Plant Base +

Avoid a deadly virus, save your health, our animals and our planet

William J Stark

Table of Contents

Introduction

"For as long as men massacre animals, they will kill each other. Indeed, he who sows the seed of murder and pain cannot reap joy and love."

Pythagoras

Do you know what it means to follow a plant-based diet? Do you want to learn the implications of a meat-based diet? Are you aware of the link between meat and several pandemics over the years? Do you want to shift to a healthier lifestyle? Are you looking for a simple diet that is easy to maintain? Do you want to do your bit for the environment? If you've answered 'yes,' to any of these questions, then you have chosen the perfect book. As you read on, you will learn in detail about the plant-based diet and how you can help to heal the earth by making the switch.

A plant-based diet might seem like an abstract concept, but in simple words, a plant-based diet is predominantly based on foods derived from plants. Making a couple of simple dietary changes is all you need to do to improve your overall health and help the environment at the same time.

Several studies and collections of research have shown various benefits of plant-based diets over the last couple of decades. From treating chronic health problems, such as diabetes to heart diseases and improving your overall health, a plant-based diet can help you in several significant ways. This is one of the reasons for its steadily increasing popularity these days.

A plant-based diet is easy to maintain and extremely sustainable. The only protocol to follow is to avoid all animal-based foods. This is the main rule you need to keep in mind, and that's about it! Depending on your overall health and fitness goals, you can customize a daily diet according to your needs and requirements.

Did you know that approximately 48% of globally available land is used for livestock farming? This industry also contributes about 18% of greenhouse gas emissions. Sadly, all of this is to derive only 18% of calories and 37% of total protein consumed by humans across the globe. These numbers are not only saddening but shocking too. It shows how easily the big meat players have turned a blind eye towards this rampant global problem.

In a study conducted by researchers at Oxford Martin School, it was noted approximately 8,000,000 human lives could be saved by 2050 if greenhouse emissions can be reduced, food production increased, and intensive animal farming reduced. Not to mention the overall health and quality of life of humans could potentially increase further due to a reduction in medical expenses of approximately $1.5 trillion (Springmann et al., 2016). These numbers sound incredible, don't they? Do you want to learn how all this could be possible? Well, a plant-based lifestyle is the answer to all these questions.

This book will show you what it means to live a plant-based lifestyle and the different benefits it offers, its overall sustainability, and various ethical considerations. Before you learn more about a plant-based lifestyle, it is important to know how it differs from a meat-oriented one.

Eating meat is not just bad for your health, but the environment too, the 'how' of it will be explained in detail in the book. Apart from this, another factor that needs to be considered is animal cruelty and the barbaric treatment animals are doled out by the meat industry. Meat production is not as sanitary as we would all like to believe. This book explores how unsafe meat production is and the harmful effects of consuming such unsafe animal products. You will also discover the link between animal products and several critical and chronic illnesses. The mad cow, Nipah virus, SARS, and the latest Covid-19 are viral illnesses and pandemics, and primarily caused due to animal products.

This book also covers in extensive detail the reality of animal agriculture. Irrespective of what the labels on food products claim, there is no such thing as ethical treatment when it comes to the big meat industry. By learning the connection between climate change, global warming, and animal farming, it will lend a new perspective to why a plant-based diet is extremely beneficial.

It is also believed a plant-based diet could be the key to ending world hunger without wreaking havoc on the environment. Once you learn about these things, it will become easier to understand why a plant-based lifestyle is sustainable and healthy.

You will read about the different ingredients and foods you can consume while on a plant-based diet, tips to transition to this new lifestyle effectively, and the common mistakes made by people who make the switch, so you can avoid them. Debunking several myths about a plant-based lifestyle will enhance your understanding of this new and healthy way of life.

Apart from all this, you will be introduced to some simple and easy plant-based recipes ideal for beginners. These recipes are both healthy and nutritious. You no longer have to spend hours sweating away in the kitchen to whip up a delicious home-cooked meal. By following these recipes, you can essentially eat your way to a better life and a healthier you.

When you learn all this, it becomes easier to transition safely to a plant-based lifestyle. You not only get a chance to improve your health but you can also do your bit for the environment. This makes a plant-based diet a win-win solution for everyone. It helps with weight loss and supports heart health; it increases energy levels, and reduces your risk of contracting certain diseases. If you are interested in improving your health or want to learn more about this intriguing lifestyle choice, you are on the right track.

Are you excited to learn more about all this? If yes, then let us get started!

Chapter One:

Why a Plant-Based Life Is Best for Your Health

A plant-based diet is believed to be one of the healthiest diets you can choose. For several years, food scientists and dieticians have been extensively discouraging the consumption of meats while reducing the intake of meat-based foods.

In this chapter, you will learn about the benefits of a plant-based diet, the harmful effects of meat, and the reasons dairy products aren't the best choice for your health.

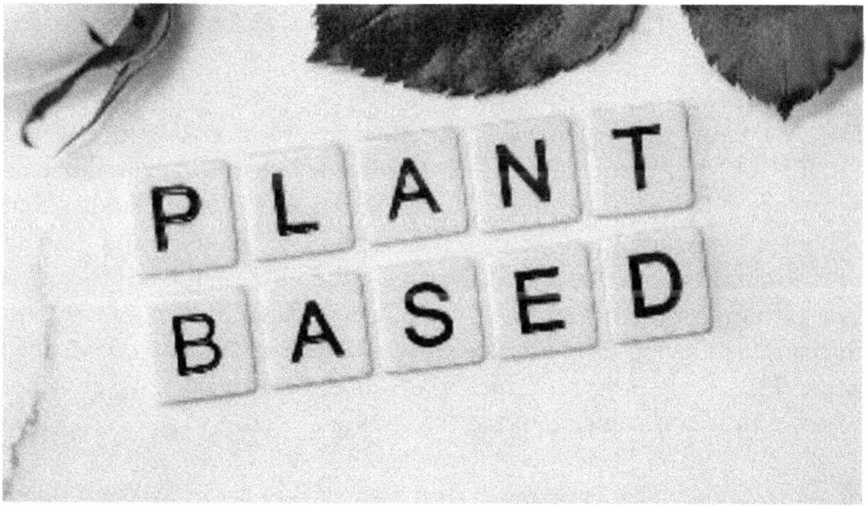

Eating Meat Makes You Sick

Eating meat is generally believed to be harmful to your health. Fatty and processed meats can make you sick. Not just meat, but different types of animal foods are unhealthy too. Foods derived directly from the animal such as flesh, and other animal produced foods are all categorized as animal foods. For instance, meat, fish, poultry, eggs, and all dairy products are all animal-based foods. Animal foods are rich in protein, but their fat content differs from one species to another. Dairy products are a great source of calcium, but they are usually unhealthy in other ways.

Red meat is quite popular, but do you know what red meat includes? All mammalian muscle meats, including but not restricted to beef, pork, veal, mutton, lamb, goat, and horse, are known as red meats.

Any meat that is salted, fermented, smoked, cured, or has undergone any other process to improve its shelf life and the overall flavor is known as processed meats. Most popular processed meats include beef and pork, but other meats include offal, poultry, or any other meat byproducts such as blood are processed meats too. Hot dogs, sausages, corned beef, beef jerky, and ham are some more examples of processed meat.

Did you know that red meat is classified as group 2-A by the World Health Organization? Group 2-A includes harmful carcinogenic substances. This classification is based on epidemiological studies that show a relationship between the consumption of red meat and the risk of colorectal cancer. Processed meats, on the other hand, are classified as a Group 1 carcinogenic. The carcinogenic classification is based on the cancer-inducing properties of an agent and not the level of risk they pose. Therefore, processed meats are in the same category as other harmful substances, including asbestos and tobacco.

An independent academic research organization known as The Global Burden of Disease Project estimated about 34,000 deaths occur across the globe annually due to cancer-inducing red meats. Not just red meats, but Cantonese style salted fish also increases the risk of nasopharyngeal cancer.

According to a study conducted by the World Cancer Research Fund (2018), there is a strong link between red meats, processed meats, dairy, and cancer. When red meat is cooked at high temperatures or is exposed to heat for prolonged periods due to various cooking processes, including grilling or barbecuing, heterocyclic amines and polycyclic aromatic hydrocarbons are formed. These substances are associated with an increased risk of colorectal cancer development according to experimental studies conducted by the same organization. Red meats also contain high levels of heme iron. Heme iron triggers the production of carcinogenic N-Nitroso compounds, which increase the risk of developing colorectal cancer.

The same logic applies to the association between processed meats and cancer. Since processed meats are cooked at high temperatures using various preservative techniques, it increases their exposure to heterocyclic amines and polycyclic aromatic hydrocarbons. The fat content in processed meats is also significantly higher than red meats, due to the synthesis of secondary bile acids. Therefore, the consumption of processed meats increases the risk of colorectal cancer.

Not just red meats and processed meats, but even dairy products can increase the risk of cancer. Dairy products are usually consumed for their high levels of calcium, but they contain other harmful substances such as lactose, casein, and residual pesticides and hormones. You will learn more about the harmful effects of dairy in the next section.

Don't get discouraged reading through these scary implications of eating meat. The good news is, the key to changing your health lies in your hands. By making a simple dietary change and following a plant-based diet, you can reduce the risk of harmful and critical illnesses, while improving your overall health and well-being.

Meat Is Not the Only Problem

To fully understand the benefits of a plant-based diet, it's important to understand why animal-based foods are harmful. Remember, animal-based foods are not just restricted to meat but include dairy too. Humans have been around for 200,000 years, but dairy became a part of our diet only about 7,500 years ago.

Dairy was not a part of the diet of an adult human and our biochemical processes are yet to catch up with this new introduction. The dairy industry's successful and intensive marketing campaigns have reinforced the idea that dairy products are good for your health. However, is there any truth to these claims? Over the years, dieticians, scientists, nutritional experts, and physicians have carefully analyzed the effect dairy has on human health and the reasons why it is not good for us.

Here are some reasons why milk and dairy products are detrimental to our health:

Truth About Organic Milk

Dairy products contain a lot of female hormones, namely estrogen and progesterone. Commercially produced dairy products are obtained from genetically engineered cows that constantly produce milk via repeated induced pregnancies. Even products labeled as 'organic' or "no hormones added" often contain high levels of these undesirable hormones. All cows, irrespective of whether they are genetically engineered or not, produce estrogen and progesterone. So, don't think you've dodged the bullet with organic milk; these hormones are present in all dairy products.

An accumulation of these hormones is undesirable for humans. Dairy consumption is a significant risk factor for all hormone-dependent malignant health conditions such as ovary, prostate, breast, uterine, and testicular cancers. Excessive intake of milk increases the levels of estrogen in humans. In men, it can result in a reduction of testosterone. According to a study conducted by Maruyama et al., (2010) childhood exposure to the external estrogen via commercial milk and dairy products can result in premature sexual maturation.

Increased Risk of Certain Diseases

Your immune system defends the body from a variety of pathogens, microbes, and other disease-causing substances. The immune system is known to attack its own cells and tissues if it loses its ability to recognize and distinguish healthy cells from the disease-inducing ones. These automatic attacks are the result of exposure to foreign particles and peptides, such as dairy products. It is believed that consumption of dairy products is directly related to the risk of autoimmune disorders.

There are two primary conditions associated with dairy's harmful effects: Type 1 diabetes and multiple sclerosis. Type 1 diabetes is also known as insulin-dependent diabetes mellitus (IDDM) or juvenile diabetes. The pancreas is attacked by the immune system, making it unable to produce insulin and regulate blood sugar levels. As per a study conducted by Dahl-Jørgensen et al., cow's milk triggers the development of IDDM. This research also suggests early exposure to cow's milk increases the risk of type 1 diabetes by 1.5 times (Dahl-Jørgensen et al., 1991).

Harmful Effects of Casein

The main protein found in dairy products is casein, and it is directly linked with the growth and development of certain types of cancer. According to a study conducted by Chan et al., (2001) on the connection between dairy and prostate cancer, the development of cancer can be regulated by reducing the levels of casein in the diet and not just the carcinogens. IGF-1 (insulin-like growth factor) is a hormone necessary for cell growth and division in regular and cancer cells. Consumption of animal protein and casein from dairy foods increases the levels of this cancer-inducing hormone.

Presence of Microorganisms

All dairy products, including milk, house a variety of microorganisms that act as carriers for foodborne pathogens. Even though these products are thoroughly sanitized via pasteurization and curing, the complete elimination of these harmful pathogens is unlikely. The most common foodborne outbreaks caused due to dairy products include salmonella, E. coli, and Listeria (Altekruse et al., 1998). The "CDC – Listeria (Listeriosis) – Outbreaks – Multistate Outbreak of Listeriosis Linked to Blue Bell Creameries Products" (2016), reports three deaths due to Listeria infections associated with Blue Bell ice creams, which were immediately recalled in April 2015.

Concentration of Pesticides

Pesticide contamination has become the new reality of modern cultivation and agriculture. This contamination affects water resources and agricultural lands needed for dairy production. Due to the high-fat content, dairy products tend to accumulate a greater proportion of these harmful pesticides. Some pesticides no longer in use, such as DDT, believed to be a human carcinogen, can still be found in the environment. These harmful pesticides make their way from the environment into the livestock and finally into the human digestive system.

Antibiotic Residue in Dairy Products

Livestock are given several antibiotics to increase their feed efficiency, growth, and to prevent infections. Antibiotic overuse leads to antibiotic resistance and leaves traces or residues of these harmful substances in the dairy products thus produced. The lack of proper record keeping of animal drug use and varying use of antibiotics from one dairy operation to another increases the risk of contamination by antibiotic residues. These residues slowly make their way from the dairy products into the human system, with damaging effects.

Detrimental to Bone Health

Years of intensive campaigning by the dairy industry has led to the popular misconception that milk is good for bone health. According to a study conducted by Weinsier et al., (2000), there is no scientific evidence to back these claims and bone health is not dependent on your dairy consumption. Numerous studies suggest that dairy consumption is actually detrimental to bone health and might also increase the risk of fractures.

Dairy products are a rich source of calcium, which deregulates the absorption and utilization of vitamin D in the body. It, in turn, harms the process of bone homeostasis. Acidosis is also induced by the high animal protein content of dairy products, which prompts the body to use calcium from its bones to neutralize the excessive acidity. Over time, a combination of these two factors harms bone health.

Going Plant-Based and Health

The "Plant-based diets: A Physician's Guide" (2016) is a detailed study of several advantages of plant-based diets. This is one of the leading reasons why practitioners across the globe are recommending a plant-based eating pattern instead of one based on animal products. A plant-based diet is not only healthy but is environment-friendly too. Therefore, it isn't surprising to note several popular celebrities such as Beyoncé and Tom Brady are staunch proponents of plant-based diets.

Irrespective of whether you are an animal lover or a nature enthusiast, a plant-based diet is one of the healthiest ways to live. Going plant-based is more of a lifestyle change than a mere shift in diet. You don't have to count calories or keep track of all the micronutrients you consume. Instead, you merely concentrate on consuming more plant-based foods while avoiding or eliminating animal-based ones.

Reduces Blood Pressure

Hypertension or high blood pressure is a health marker of various serious illnesses such as cardiovascular diseases, Type II diabetes, and strokes. The good news is there are different foods you can consume to help regulate and lower your blood pressure. According to a study published in JAMA internal medicine, and analysis data obtained from 39 studies, low levels of blood pressure were observed in those who followed omnivorous diets (Yokoyama et al., 2014). Compared to nonvegetarians, vegetarians had a 34% lower risk of developing hypertension, according to a study conducted by Chuang et al., in 2016.

Better Cardiovascular Health

Animal products, especially meats, are filled with saturated fats that increase the risk of cardiovascular disorders when consumed in excess. By avoiding meat and increasing your intake of plant-based foods, this condition can be effectively reversed. According to (Caulfield et al., 2019) plant-based diets are associated with a lower risk of cardiovascular disease related mortality in middle aged adults. A plant-based diet reduces the risk of cardiovascular diseases by 16% and mortality due to this condition by 31%. To make the most of the benefits offered by a plant-based diet, it is important to pay attention to the ingredients you consume. Loading up on healthy plant-based foods such as olive oil, fruits, vegetables, legumes, and whole grains is always better than increasing your intake of refined grains and sugary processed foods.

Reduces the Risk of Diabetes

There exists an undeniable relationship between Type 2 diabetes and diet. Weight is also an important risk factor because the accumulation of fatty tissues makes the cells insulin resistant. A study on a plant-based diet and Type 2 diabetes suggests the risk of developing Type 2 diabetes can be reduced by almost 34% by consuming a plant-based diet consisting of high-quality plant foods (Satija et al., 2016). Unlike animal foods, plant-based foods have low levels of saturated fats. Reducing saturated fats can lower your cholesterol levels and thereby reduce the risk of Type 2 diabetes as well. Only 2.9% of vegans had Type 2 diabetes, while it was as high as 7.6% in nonvegetarians as per a study conducted on diet and prevalence of diabetes by Tonstad (2009).

Weight Loss and Management

A plant-based diet drastically reduces the risk of obesity. Even if weight loss is not your priority, you can easily provide your body all the nourishment it needs and enhance your overall health by increasing your intake of healthy and wholesome plant-based foods. A substantial difference between the health of meat-eaters and non meat-eaters was a result of their eating habits. The mean BMI for meat-eaters was found to be 28.8, while the BMI for vegans was at 23.6, which is within the regular BMI range for adults.

Based on a 2017 study, 65 overweight adults managed to lose 9.25 pounds on an average when they followed a plant-based diet for a year. The primary reason for weight loss is the low glycemic index of different whole grains, fruits, and vegetables (Wright et al., 2017).

Foods with a low glycemic index take longer to digest and promote a feeling of satiety. It, in turn, naturally decreases your appetite without making you feel you are following a restrictive eating pattern. Once you consume foods rich in complex carbs, dietary fibers, and healthy fats, your overall calorie intake reduces naturally. A calorie deficit is incredibly important for weight loss. It occurs only when your calorie intake is less than your energy expenditure. When combined with sufficient exercise, a plant-based diet promotes weight loss and makes it easier to maintain this weight loss.

A Longer Life

According to research conducted by (Kim et al., 2019) a plant-based diet helps to reduce mortality rate by about 25%. This is perhaps one of the most significant (and certainly dramatic) benefits of a plant-based diet. This effect can be further enhanced by up to 5% by increasing your intake of healthy and wholesome plant foods and reducing the consumption of processed foods according to a study. By increasing your intake of healthy plant foods such as whole grains, vegetables, fruits, and reducing the intake of sodas, sugary treats, and other processed foods, you can ensure your body gets all the nourishment it needs without bogging it down with dangerous additives and empty calories.

Reduces the Risk of Cancer

According to the American Institute of Cancer Research, the simplest way to obtain cancer-protective essential nutrients is by consuming a plant-based diet filled with fresh vegetables, whole grains, fruits, and legumes. These ingredients contain fiber, phytochemicals, vitamins, minerals, and various antioxidants that offer cancer-protective properties. As mentioned in the previous sections, several animal-based products contain cancer-causing agents. By eliminating these items from your diet, you can reduce your risk of cancer.

Better Energy Levels

Plant-based foods are rich in antioxidants, dietary fibers, minerals, and vitamins. A combination of all these things makes you feel full and satisfied and gives your body all the nutrients it needs. Even if you are worried you are not getting the required nutrients, there are various vegan substitutes readily available to fill in any gaps.

By paying a little attention to your diet and going through the list of essential nutrients discussed in the subsequent chapters, you can optimize your body's overall health and energy levels. A plant-based diet will make you feel more energetic than a predominantly meat-based one. For instance, how do you feel after eating a 6-ounce steak? Probably heavy and lethargic, am I right? Now, how would you feel after eating a bowl of salad? You will feel lighter after eating those greens. So, your energy levels will improve, and post-meal energy slumps will decrease.

Myths About Plant-Based Diets

In a culture predominantly made of omnivores, vegans and vegetarians are widely misunderstood. Not only are they grossly misunderstood, but they are also the unintended victims of several misconceptions. In this section, let's debunk some of those misconceptions about plant-based diets. Debunking these myths and learning the facts will strengthen your understanding about a plant-based diet so you feel confident about your transition.

Myth #1: Plant-Based Diets Are Deficient in Protein

A popular misconception is that plant-based diets don't offer sufficient protein. The most common sources of protein are often animal-based, and hence the misconception. Unsurprisingly, almost every vegan or vegetarian would have heard the irritating question "But, where do you get your protein?" The notion that plant-based diets are inherently lacking in protein is nothing more than a misconception. There are several plant-based and healthy sources of proteins, such as vegetables, grains, and fruits. Also, soy products, such as tofu are especially rich in protein. Other healthy, plant-based proteins you can add to your diet include quinoa, tempeh, spirulina, edamame, lentils, peanuts, almonds, and chickpeas. You don't have to depend on animal foods to derive the protein your body needs. There are plenty of plant-based alternatives to choose from to keep both your palate happy and your body satisfied.

Myth #2: Honey Is Vegan

Honeybees make honey. A plant-based diet excludes everything derived from animals. This myth is based on a misconception that honey bees naturally secrete honey, but honey bees secrete honey for their consumption. How mammals produce milk to feed their young ones, honey is a form of sustenance for bees. In fact, all the honey produced by bees in a hive is their winter storage.

Drastic industrialization and excessive commercialization, coupled with increased consumption of honey, has reduced the global bee population. Pollination is a vital process and has a direct effect on the overall ecosystem. It is important for the growth of all plants and crops. Without bees, pollination takes a backseat. This is a fair reason to stop using honey. Honey can be easily replaced with any other plant-based sweetener, and doing so would be in humanity's best interest.

Myth #3: Soy Milk Is The Only Available Alternative

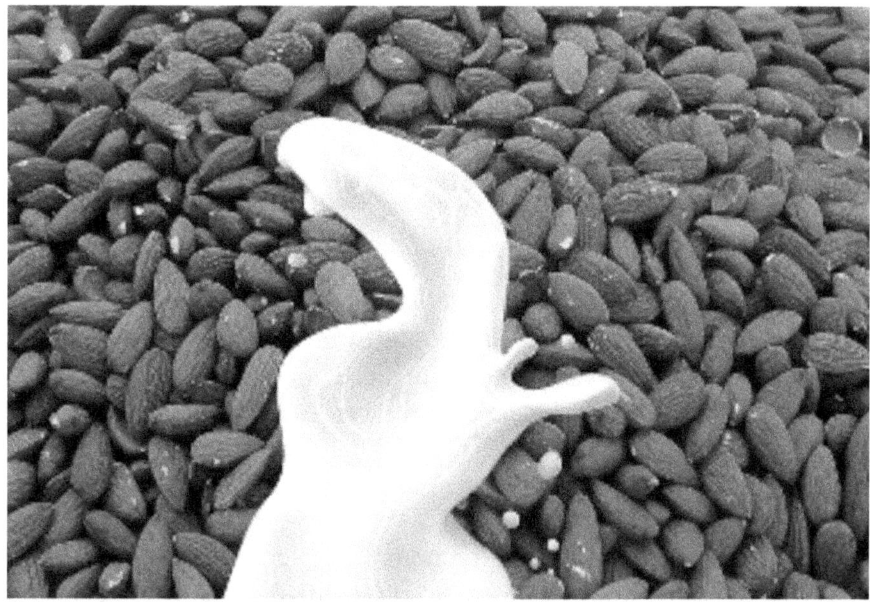

The growing awareness about the benefits of a plant-based diet has introduced several alternatives for dairy products. These days dairy substitutes are not only readily available but are healthy, too. A lot of people often believe soymilk is the only available alternative for regular milk. Well, there are several types of nut-based milk and other plant-based milk available in the market. For instance, hazelnut milk, almond milk, rice milk, oat milk, coconut milk, and hemp milk are just a few of the non-dairy substitutes you can try. You can also look for vegan dairy products fortified with vitamin D, B12, and other vital nutrients.

Myth #4: Soy Protein Increases Estrogen

Estrogen comes in different forms, and it is not all the same. There is a difference between plant-based and animal-based estrogen. Plant-based estrogen is known as a phytoestrogen, and it isn't harmful. It is good for women and is believed to reduce the risk of breast cancer. Another misconception is that consumption of soy protein reduces the production of testosterone in men. Isoflavones present in soy products might bind with similar receptors as estrogen, but they aren't the same. Therefore, it is unfair to wrongly assume soy proteins increase the production of estrogen in men.

Myth #5: No Dairy Products = No Calcium

As mentioned in the earlier section, dairy is harmful to human health. The dairy industry would have you believe milk and dairy products are the only sources of calcium. Their widespread and intensive marketing and advertising campaigns have convinced millions of people across the globe to believe they would keel over from weak bones if they don't get their quota of dairy. There is hardly any truth to back up these claims.

Dairy products contain a certain amount of calcium, but they are high in cholesterol, saturated fats, and several contaminants. Adding such a harmful collection to your daily diet doesn't make any sense. There are many other better sources of calcium, and none are animal-based. For instance, dark leafy green vegetables such as collard greens, mustard greens, Swiss chard, broccoli, all types of legumes, organic soy foods, and almonds are loaded with calcium. These days, you can even find varieties of calcium-fortified vegan milk too. Instead of putting dairy cows through a life of misery, finding plant-based alternatives is humane and merciful—and delicious!

Myth #6: Plants Feel Pain

The usual argument meat-eaters make about a plant-based diet is that plants also feel pain. If plants feel pain, then shouldn't eating them be as bad as eating meat? Well, this is what they would want you to believe. However, they couldn't be further from the truth. To start with, plants don't have a central nervous system, neurons, or a brain, unlike animals. When it comes to following a plant-based diet, we must draw a line somewhere. We all need to eat to survive and sustain ourselves. We have the choice t0 determine where this food comes from. Eating plants is better than feeding them to other animals and slaughtering these animals for our food requirements. Plucking a fruit off the tree is similar to clipping a nail! That said, I think we can all agree, slaughtering an animal would go beyond trimming your nails.

Myth #7: Veganism Causes Nutrient Deficiencies

"Dairy is the only source of calcium."

"There are no plant-based proteins."

"A plant-based diet is filled with carbs and has no nutrients."

These are some common misconceived comments and misunderstandings, which have led to the belief that a plant-based diet leads to severe nutritional deficiencies. Plant foods are rich in complex carbohydrates, dietary fats, proteins, and various micronutrients. As long as you eat a healthy and well-balanced diet, you don't have to worry about nutritional deficiencies. Even if you are worried, there are different plant-based supplements you can add to your daily diet to ensure your body gets nourished. You will learn more about those in the subsequent chapters.

Myth #8: All Plant Foods Are Good

One myth a lot of people believe is all plant foods are good. Remember, all plant foods are not created equally; some are more nutritious than others. Some foods should be avoided altogether, even if they are plant-based. Take a moment and think about it. What do you think is healthier, eating French fries or munching on raw carrots and cauliflower? Both are plant-based, but one is clearly healthier than another.

As mentioned in the previous section, there are several advantages of a plant-based diet. From improving your overall health to losing weight and feeling more energetic, the gains are seemingly endless with a plant-based diet. A simple rule you can follow to ensure that your body gets all the nutrients it needs is to include different types of colorful foods to your daily meals. Remember to eat the rainbow, because foods of different colors represent different nutrients present within.

Before you purchase any prepackaged or processed food, carefully go through the list of ingredients. Look for any artificial additives, chemicals, refined sugars and flours, and preservatives it contains. If there are any ingredients mentioned that you wouldn't use in your kitchen or cannot identify, stay away from such food options. The more artificial ingredients the food contains, the less healthy and more processed it is. A plant-based diet is not restrictive. There are different options available, which you will learn more about later. It is truly a well-balanced and incredibly diverse diet.

Myth #9: Plant-Based Diets Are Expensive

A plant-based diet doesn't have to be expensive. It's time to let go of any misconceptions you probably have about the costs involved. It's all about the choices you make. For instance, it *would* blow a hole in your pocket if you splurge on turmeric lattes and smoothies from the chic vegan café every morning, opt for prepackaged organic foods, or constantly eat out. If you continue these eating habits, it will soon become expensive.

As with any other diet, it's all about your conscious choices and decisions that determine the costs involved. Let's look at a more sensible alternative to the plant-based choices made in the above example. If you are willing to cook most of your meals at home, it will significantly reduce your food expenses. Likewise, instead of splurging on processed and packaged plant-based foods, try to make these snacks at home. If improving your health is a priority, forgo all sorts of processed foods and replace them with healthy, raw, and wholesome ingredients. Follow the simple plant-based recipes given in this book, and you can reduce your food budget in no time!

Myth 10: A Plant-Based Diet Will Make Me Tired/Hungry

Your body needs a variety of nutrients. As long as you provide it all the nutrients it needs, it will function at its optimal level. You don't have to worry about feeling tired or hungry while following a plant-based diet. Pay attention to the different macros you consume and be mindful of the diet you follow. If you replace all processed ingredients with healthy and wholesome ones, it will make you feel energetic. Give your body some time to get used to the new diet, so you can see the benefits it offers.

Chapter Two:

Pandemics, Novel Viruses, and the Link to Meat

Consuming animal products is extremely unhealthy, but it isn't the only thing that harms the world. Even the production and farming processes have become the leading causes of several critical health conditions and diseases. Blame it on the poor hygiene or widespread unethical practices but several worldwide health disasters such as the bird flu, the mad cow disease, or even the latest Covid-19 crisis are associated with animal products.

All these diseases have spread from animals to humans, but the only ones to be blamed here are humans. Our increasing demand for meat from different animals such as turkeys, pigs, chickens, cows, and other exotic wildlife is a primary reason for the hefty price humanity has to pay.

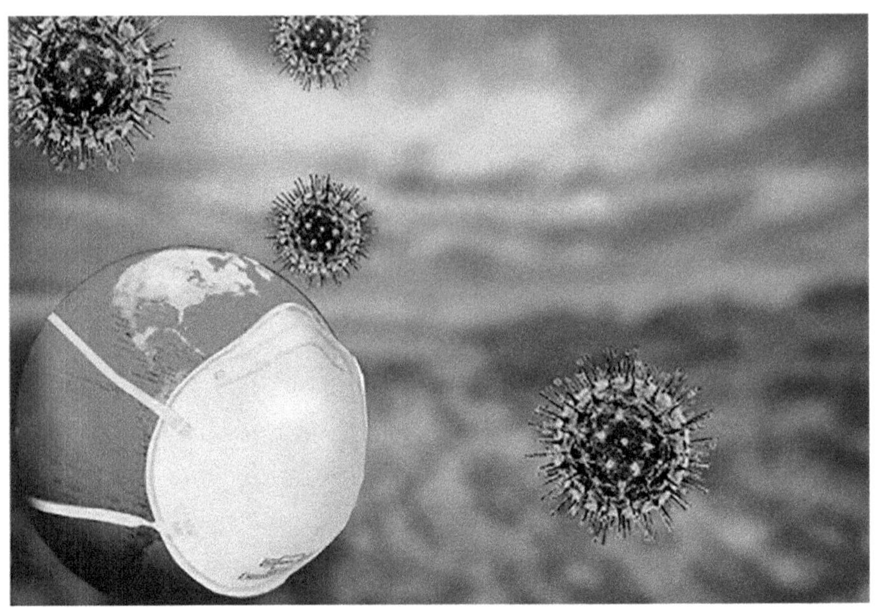

Brief Timeline of Infectious Diseases

The production of food, especially with an animal origin, has contributed to several outbreaks of various infectious diseases over the years. Let us look at some severe infections that spread from animals to humans.

1918 Influenza Pandemic

One of the most severe pandemics humanity has had to deal with was the 1918 outbreak of influenza. This pandemic was caused by a variant of an H1N1 virus strain. This strain was believed to have genes of avian origin. The influenza outbreak became a pandemic because of how quickly it spread. Its spread was associated with the troop movements and overcrowding due to WW1. The situation further worsened due to the lack of a viable vaccine, treatment, and the high vulnerability of healthy young adults. According to the CDC, it caused 50 million deaths across the globe of which 675,000 were reported within the United States alone.

The first instance of this viral outbreak was reported at Camp Funston, Kansas where over 100 soldiers showed flu-like symptoms. The symptoms of this flu included chills, tiredness, fever, and all the usual symptoms of the common flu. The numbers quintupled within a week. The properties of this specific strain of H1N1 virus weren't fully understood despite its overall devastation. The outbreak wasn't restricted to the United States, and cases were reported in parts of Europe and Asia too. During the same year, there was a second and deadlier wave of the same strain of influenza with high rates of mortality. The 1918 influenza pandemic is known as the Spanish Flu because Spain was the worst hit nation. The exact cause of this virus and its transmission to humans is still unknown. That said, it is known that strains of influenza viruses are common in birds and pigs. Some believe this virus could have been passed on to humans from infected pigs.

Mad Cow Disease

Bovine spongiform encephalopathy (BSE) is commonly known as mad cow disease. This is a fatal disease that targets the central nervous system of adult cattle and is highly transmissible. It regresses slowly and is degenerative. The first noted case of the mad cow disease appeared in the 1970s. Initially, it was believed to be caused by prions that cause scrapie in sheep.

The first cases were brushed away as isolated incidents before the world realized it was in for a brutal shock. The first outbreak occurred in 1986 in the United Kingdom. This disease is named such because of the unnatural behavior displayed by the cattle. By 1988, more than 400 cattle were diagnosed with BSE in Britain. Due to the spread of this disease, a ban on human consumption of certain types of organ meats, the brain, and spinal cord obtained from cattle was implemented.

The United States also prohibited the import of goats, cattle, sheep, and bison and other live livestock from other countries that reported BSE. During the early 90s, Britain declared there was no threat to humans from this disease. In January 1993, more than a thousand new cases started to appear every week in the United Kingdom.

From then until 2010, more than 184,5000 BSE cases were confirmed in the UK. Testing and extensive research showed an association between a prion induced disease in humans known as Creutzfeldt-Jakob disease (vCJD), which was first reported in 1996 after the BSE outbreak.

The primary cause of the spread of this disease in humans was the consumption of beef products contaminated by the disease-inducing prion. Consuming the nervous system tissue, such as the spinal cord and the brain of any cattle infected with this disease, triggered the spread in humans. It's not just the United States and the United Kingdom that reported this disease, but it was confirmed in several other countries across the globe. Austria, Finland, Belgium, Italy, Czech Republic, Denmark, Japan, France, Luxembourg, Poland, Slovakia, Slovenia, Spain, Switzerland, Portugal, Ireland, are some of the countries that reported cases.

This degenerative disease not only affects individuals of all age groups, but it is tricky to diagnose until it's too late. During the early stages of vCJD, the reported symptoms include depression and reduction in coordination. As it starts to progress, it triggers the onset of dementia and is usually considered fatal.

The Nipah Virus Infection

A member of the Paramyxoviridae viruses, the Nipah virus (NiV), was first identified in 1999 in Malaysia and Singapore. There was a sudden outbreak of respiratory illnesses and encephalitis among pig farmers and all those who worked in close contact with pigs in 1999. The first case was registered in a small village named Sungai Nipah in Malaysia.

It was reported several pig farmers contracted encephalitis. This virus was initially believed to be related to the Hendra virus commonly associated with bat species, which was immediately singled out. However, it was later identified that fruit bats or flying foxes belonging to the Pteropus genus were the primary carriers.

There is some evidence that shows this infection among various domesticated animals such as horses, dogs, goats, and sheep could be infected by the NiV virus. The research revealed this virus is present naturally in the urine, feces, saliva, and other bodily fluids of fruit bats. It's speculated that various deforestation programs in the Malaysian peninsula where the pig farms were situated had fruit trees, which attracted these bats from their natural habitat to human locations.

This exposed domestic pigs to bat feces and urine. All these excretions and secretions triggered the infections in pigs. The practice of intensive pig farming led to the rapid and rampant spread of this infection even before the authorities could take steps to prevent or contain it. Due to the intense farming activities, all those who came in contact with the infected pigs also contracted this deadly infection.

This virus is classified as a zoonotic disease. Any disease caused by pathogens spread between animals and humans is known as such. According to the incident report in Malaysia and Singapore, the transmission from pigs to humans was via direct contact with the secretions or the excretions from infected animals. There were also reports of this deadly outbreak in Bangladesh. The primary carriers in Bangladesh were believed to be bats. There was no intermediate host involved. It was identified that the consumption of raw palm sap and climbing trees contaminated and covered with bat excrement led to human transmission of this disease.

The primary symptoms of this infection include fever, drowsiness, headaches, disorientation, confusion, and in later stages, it can result in a coma. In some instances, it proved fatal. During this deadly outbreak in Malaysia, approximately 50% of all the clinically apparent human transmission cases were fatal. However, it presents itself as different symptoms in infected animals. It manifests as a respiratory and neurologic syndrome and is quite contagious. The clinical signs tend to vary depending on the age of the animal and its living conditions.

The NiV outbreak is another example of the lapses in intensive animal rearing and the apparent flaws in the existing system. The lack of proper sanitation and necessary precautions coupled with unhygienic living conditions of pigs triggered its spread.

SARS Outbreak

SARS stands for Severe Acute Respiratory Syndrome. It is a type of coronavirus known as SARS-associated coronavirus (SARS-COV) and is a viral respiratory illness. The first case of SARS was reported in Asia in 2003. Though it was reported in February, this viral illness quickly spread across the globe within a few months. From Europe to North America, South America and most of Asia were contaminated by the global SARS outbreak. During the 2003 outbreak, according to the data gathered by the World Health Organization (WHO), around 8,000 people became sick and over 700 deaths were reported. Before the authorities finally managed to contain it, this disease spread to over 24 countries.

The symptoms of SARS include a high fever of more than 100.4°F, headaches, body aches, and a general feeling of discomfort. At the onset, the infected individuals might experience mild respiratory symptoms and even pneumonia in some instances. Person-to-person contact is how this disease spreads. The respiratory droplets from an infected person's sneeze or cough can infect others. This virus can also spread if the infected person touches any objects or surfaces and contaminates them with infectious pathogens. These symptoms can take anywhere between 2 to 7 days to appear after contact with an infected person or an animal.

As with the previous outbreaks, even SARS is a zoonotic disease. It is believed this virus probably originated in wild bats. After this, it probably spread to civets and other similar mammals. The virus kept mutating while it transmitted and adapted itself in various animals until it started infecting humans. There were several opportunities for this deadly virus to come into contact with humans. In some areas of Asia, bats are often used as food. Traditional folk medicine sometimes calls for bat feces. The musk obtained from the scent glands of civets found in Africa and Asia is used to create perfumes. In some parts of the globe, civets are hunted for their meat and believed to be delicacies. Even if SARS was not the result of intensive animal farming practices, it was caused by the human demand for wild animals, meat, and other byproducts.

Avian Influenza or the Bird Flu

Avian Influenza is also known as bird flu. The first recorded outbreak of the bird flu occurred in 2004. This viral infection not only infects birds, as the name suggests, but also spreads to humans and other animals. The most common type of bird flu virus is H5N1. Even though this virus was first discovered in 1997, according to the World Health Organization WHO the outbreak didn't occur until 2004.

As per WHO, the mortality rate of H5N1 infected humans is up to 60%. There isn't any scientific evidence to prove this virus spreads due to human-to-human contact. It presents itself with usual flu-like symptoms such as diarrhea, respiratory difficulties, fever of 100.4°F, muscle aches, sore throat, cough, and a runny nose.

There are various types of bird flu, but the H5N1 is the only avian Influenza that has infected humans. The first infection was reported in Hong Kong in 1997, and it was linked with handling infected poultry. It usually occurs in wild aquatic birds, but can be contracted by domestic poultry too. This virus spreads if humans come in contact with the feces and bodily secretions from the nose, mouth, and eyes of the infected birds. With research, it was notified more than a hundred different species of wild birds had avian Influenza A viruses. Gulls, shorebirds, terns and other aquatic birds such as ducks, swans, and geese are believed to be hosts for avian influenza viruses.

Even domesticated species such as chickens and turkeys can be infected with this virus. If these species come in contact with the infected waterfowls, they can contract the virus directly or indirectly. Indirect contamination occurs when the domesticated birds come in contact with surfaces contaminated by the wild species. It is difficult to detect this infection in poultry because it presents itself as mild signs. The most common signs are ruffled feathers and a reduction in egg production.

In intensive farming practices, especially poultry, the birds are housed in tightly packed cages. Even a single infected bird can easily contaminate an entire farm. The lack of proper sanitation and regular maintenance, coupled with poor housing conditions, are some factors that led to the rapid spread of this virus.

Another factor to be considered is the lack of veterinary care in the meat industry. The common symptoms of avian Influenza are difficult to detect. The usual practice in this industry is to slaughter any animal, which no longer proves to be useful. Therefore, the chances of unknowingly sending the infected flocks to slaughterhouses are quite high. It is believed, the mortality rate of this avian Influenza is between 90-100% and can prove to be fatal within 48-hours in chickens.

Swine Flu

The H1N1 virus or the swine flu virus is a type of influenza virus. The symptoms it causes are quite similar to the regular flu. As its name suggests, this virus originated in pigs, but slowly spread to humans. Once human contact was achieved, it easily spread from one individual to another. The H1N1 outbreak occurred in 2009 and is one of the most contagious diseases known to humankind.

In August 2010, it was declared as a pandemic by the WHO. H1N1 is contagious and is believed to spread like other strains of flu. The flu shot developed every year by the Centers For Disease Control And Prevention includes vaccination against the H1N1 virus. Therefore, the simplest way to deal with this pandemic is to prevent it. Since it originates from pigs, it's important to look at the meat industry once again. According to the CDC, the fatality total of the pandemic swine flu was 575,400.

The H1N1 virus is a type A influenza virus. These viruses possess an innate ability to mix with other viral strains creating a novel strain. This is what happened during the H1N1 outbreak in 2009. Pigs are known to contract three different types of influenza—human, swine, and avian. Therefore, they are the perfect hosts and carriers that allow viruses to mix and mutate into new strains.

The H1N1 virus genes consist of human, swine, and avian strains, which were metamorphosed in pigs and hence the name swine flu. Influenza is common among pigs, and most pigs contact it at some point or the other during the winter. At times, this virus can be transmitted from pigs to humans who come in contact with them. This is believed to be the primary factor responsible for the transmission of H1N1.

When humans contract this virus, it reacts the same way any flu does. It is an airborne illness that can contaminate different surfaces. It can also be transmitted from one person to another through infected droplets in the air.

Ebola Virus

EVD or the Ebola virus disease is a fatal viral infection that has flared up in repeated outbreaks on the African continent. Primates such as gorillas, chimpanzees, and monkeys, as well as humans are the most common targets of this virus. This virus was discovered for the first time in 1976, near the Ebola River in Congo, leading to its namesake. The primary cause of this virus is still unclear. Still, given the similar nature of other viral infections transferred from animals, the most likely sources include bats and other nonhuman primates. This virus spreads to humans when they come in contact with blood and other body fluids secreted by an infected animal. Once a human being contracts it, it can easily spread in a community.

This harmful virus can cause severe bleeding, organ failure, and death. The Ebola outbreak between 2014-2016 in West Africa started in southeastern Guinea, which later spread to urban areas and ultimately became a pandemic. As with all the other genetic diseases, this too, was caused when humans came in contact with wild animals. Consuming meat from wild animals or bush meat is not only unsafe it is illegal in several countries across the globe.

The Covid-19 Pandemic

With a rise in the human population, there's been a significant increase in the demand for meat and animal products as well. This change has cost humanity dearly. Pandemics have become more frequent than they ever were. Do you see the correlation?

The latest addition to the long list of deadly pandemics is the Covid-19 or the Novel Coronavirus. Coronavirus is the name used to describe a group of viruses that are known to cause diseases in humans and animals. For instance, SARS is caused by a strain of coronavirus. When compared with the SARS pandemic of 2002, the COVID pandemic is considered worse. The new strain of the coronavirus reported for the first time in 2019 results in severe acute respiratory syndrome. Since it was discovered in 2019, it is known as Covid-19.

On March 11, 2019, the World Health Organization declared coronavirus to be a global pandemic. Within a few months, this virus spread across various nations and has effectively managed to cripple a vast number of economies. In six months, this virus affected millions of people across the globe and resulted in a significant death count, unlike any occurrence known to modern humanity. This is believed to be the deadliest pandemic.

Coronavirus is quite common in certain species of animals, such as camels and bats. However, the transmission of these viruses from animals to humans was rare and almost unknown until 2019. It isn't clear how the virus actually spreads from animals to humans, but there are several theories. According to the WHO, the coronavirus is a rather large family of different viruses, including the ones that cause the common cold to severe respiratory diseases, such as the Middle East Respiratory Syndrome and Severe Acute Respiratory Syndrome.

Initial reports suggest the first case reporting the spread of the novel coronavirus from animals to humans occurred in Wuhan. Wuhan is a small province in China and is believed to be ground zero of the coronavirus pandemic. The Huanan seafood market located in Wuhan is believed to be the possible source of this virus.

The usual suspects of the coronavirus include exotic wild animals, bats, and snakes. The unhealthy practices in the meat and poultry industries harm the environment and are a health hazard. Even if you overlook the unethical treatment of animals, you cannot miss their failure to ensure animal meats' safety. The Huanan seafood wholesale market is a wet market. Wet markets are quite similar to farmers' markets where fresh produce is displayed.

In these markets, some stalls sell fresh seafood, live exotic animals, meat, and other living creatures that could be consumed by humans. These markets also sell bush meat, which is illegal in most countries across the world. For instance, the Huanan wet market has a live section, where animals from different species are slaughtered and made readily available for sale.

The most common species available are baby crocodiles, snakes, beavers, and even porcupines. These markets are known as wet markets because of all the flowing liquid from the melting ice used to keep the meat cold, organs and blood from slaughtered animals, and the tubs of water used to store the live fish.

When animals and birds are forced to live in tightly packed, high-stress environments and watch one another being killed, it creates undesirable reactions within the animal. Since this seems to be common in the meat industry, it is unsurprising that most of the animal products available in the market are obtained from unhealthy practices. It further worsens the health implications because of the various antimicrobial resistance and foodborne diseases triggered by the overuse of antibiotics in the meat industry.

It's not just the wet markets that are proving to be breeding grounds for deadly viruses, it is important to look at wildlife markets too. Even if illegal, these are prevalent in several countries. The wildlife markets sell wild animals for their meat or as domesticated pets. It's not only difficult to track these establishments, but controlling them has become almost impossible. Most of this trafficking is conducted on secret underground networks or the dark web. The World Wildlife Fund conducted a survey in April that showed that 93% of participants in Hong Kong, Myanmar, Japan, Thailand, and Vietnam were in favor of eliminating all illegal and unregulated wildlife and wet markets.

In response to the outbreak of the deadly disease, all wet markets were closed for a while in China. However, all these measures came a little too late. By then, the deadly virus had spread across the globe and had several nations in its clutches. This virus single-handedly managed to send nearly the entire world into a lockdown.

The common symptoms of Covid-19 are headache, breathlessness, fever, sore throat, cough, chills, muscle pain, and loss of smell or taste. The virus can take anywhere from 2 to 14 days to incubate, and the same stands true for these symptoms to appear.

Instead of blaming animals for the outbreak, it would be better to look at the human operations that led to it. The civilized thing to do is closely examine the trade of animal meat. Animals are not only housed in inhumane conditions, but the workers are treated no better. The lack of proper medical facilities and personnel, congested spaces, and the absence of regulations are the leading causes of the spread of rampant diseases and illnesses.

All these outbreaks and pandemics are primarily caused due to the human demand for animal meats and products. The ever-growing demand for animal foods forces the animal farming industries to commercialize their operations, cut corners, and make several unnecessary compromises. The lack of ethical practices, absence of strict laws, low or no maintenance, and improper handling of animals are some of the apparent causes of the spread of severe illnesses from animals to humans. In the end, humans are the ones paying the hefty price of their unreasonable demands.

The latest Covid-19 pandemic is proof of the direct link between meat and viral infections.

Chapter Three:

The Cruelty of Animal Agriculture

Even if a majority of Americans believe animal foods are sourced humanely, it's not the reality. Annually more than ten billion land-based animals and countless aquatic species are purely raised with the intent of food farming and almost all of these animals survive in unacceptable conditions.

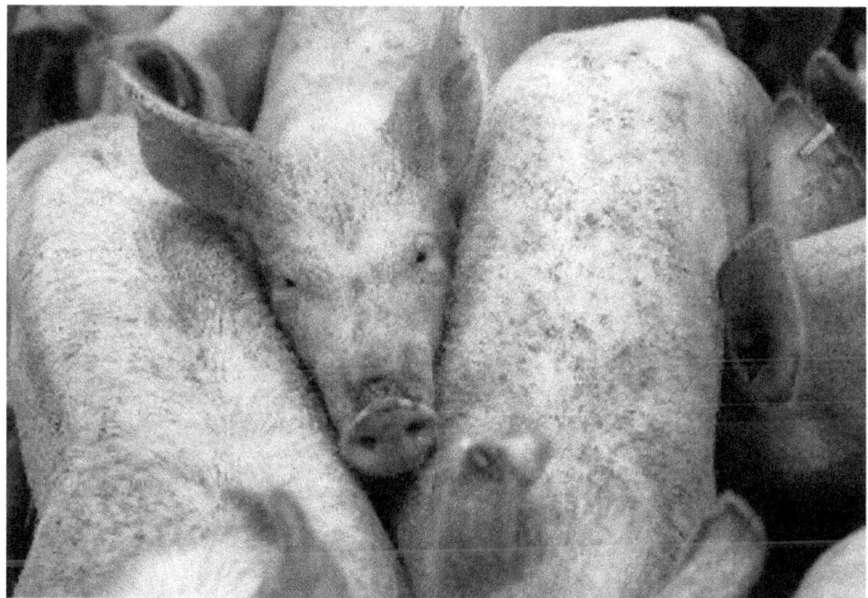

Common Misconceptions About Food Labels

Specific terms often appear on packages of eggs, meat, and dairy products, which are believed to be an indicator of the animal welfare standards. In reality, most of these terms are either not defined by the law or are used loosely. Customers don't want to buy the seemingly expensive products because they are unsure of what the terms really mean. It, in turn, adversely affects all those who truly raise animals, placing animal-welfare goals above everything else. Before learning more about animal agriculture and cruelty, it is essential to understand what different terms on packages mean. Here are the most widely misunderstood food labels.

Natural

A label bearing the term natural is often believed to signify no adverse effect on the animal's welfare. If an animal is raised purely for slaughter and in horrible living conditions, what is natural about it?

Free-Range

Free-range eggs are quite common these days. Walk into your local supermarket, and you will undoubtedly find some "free-range" eggs. Did you know the term free-range has no legal definition whatsoever when used for animal products such as dairy, eggs, pork, or beef? If there is no legal definition, this term is once again quite subjective. The idea of animal welfare is rendered redundant due to such haphazard use of these terms. It might momentarily assuage a buyer's conscience, but it does nothing for the animals.

USDA Organic

This label might make a consumer feel confident about the humane treatment of animals, or how the animal food was sourced. It's nothing more than a vague and poorly enforced regulation dictated for animal rearing. It doesn't include any rules associated with slaughter or transport of such animals.

Humanely Raised

As with free-range, there is no legal definition of the phrase "raised humanely." Without a proper definition, these terms are somewhat subjective due to the lack of qualified standards.

Cage-Free

A lot of consumers wrongly believe cage-free animal products signify the humane treatment and housing of animals. This label merely means the animals were not raised in cages. This is a clever play on words, especially in terms of poultry meats. Meat birds are seldom raised in cages and are instead housed in tightly packed and overcrowded sheds.

Hormone-Free

Hormone-free or no added hormones are not a label approved by the law when used for poultry or pigs. It usually only refers to synthetically administered hormones, leaving out other key areas of animal transport, care, and eventual placement in the supermarket. Therefore, any animal food, which bears this label is rather meaningless.

Now that you've gone through these terms, do these labels mean something different to you? Perhaps you're feeling a bit defeated and deceived. The good news is, you have the power to stop animal cruelty.

Unless you understand the real meaning of such food labels, making informed decisions becomes incredibly tricky. Most of these terms are often coined by the big players in the animal food industry who are trying to factor in their paychecks at the expense of animals.

Loopholes in Laws

Laws are enforced with the notion of protecting or preventing certain acts. Therefore, it is but natural to assume the existing laws enacted within the United States were created with the intent of protecting farm animals and dictating humane guidelines for animal rearing. Sadly, reality is startling and unsettling. Chilling statistics show animals raised purely for food are the least protected animals anywhere. Let's take a look at the loopholes in the existing laws.

Federal Laws

There are no specific federal laws that protect animals living on farms. Two laws are implemented concerning the transport and slaughter of farm animals. However, these laws don't include any poultry species that account for a vast chunk of land animals slaughtered.

Any farm animals that are transported across the state lines through modes other than air or water must be unloaded after every 28 hours for food, water, and for rest. However, this law is riddled with loopholes that are thoroughly exploited. The lack of proper enforcement and paltry fines further increases the violations. For instance, this law doesn't apply to farm animals that are transported through air or water. Though most farm animals are transported via modes of land transportation, some instances are outside the purview of this law.

All livestock have to be rendered insensible to pain and suffering before slaughter, according to the provisions of The Humane Methods Of Livestock Slaughter Act. A blatant loophole of this law is that it doesn't include poultry. Poultry forms a majority of animal food, and there are no laws to grant them humane treatment. Different forms of religious slaughter such as halal or kosher are also exempted from the premise of this law.

State Laws

Since federal laws don't offer any protection to these helpless animals, state laws are believed to be their defense. Unfortunately, most of the state laws in the US exempt farm animals or certain types of farm animals from anti-cruelty provisions. The meager protections available under state laws become redundant because of such blatant exemptions. Even if some states have farm animals in their list of anti-cruelty laws, they are seldom enforced. The lack of laws or absence of their enforcement, even when in place, don't offer farm animals any protection.

Anti-whistleblower bills or Ag-Gag laws are being incorporated into several state legislatures. These laws might seem reasonable at first glance, but they aren't designed to protect farm animals. They are designed to merely protect the big corporations from being exposed for their inhumane treatment of animals. Ideally, animal abuse should be deemed illegal. Instead, these laws are created with the notion of illegalizing the exposure, documentation, and reporting of such abuse. The laws created to protect the farm animals seemingly are weaponized against them to line the pockets of big meat players.

States are also pushing bills for the enactment of The Farm Act and laws. The livestock industry is supposed to reform all inhumane and destructive practices. Instead, they are pushing for bills that reduce the state's control over their prohibitive practices. Once these laws are in place, states will have no power whatsoever to criminalize the cruel confinement of innocent farm animals.

There seems to be a silver lining because a lot of states are implementing bans on confinement. It essentially prohibits extreme modes of confining farm animals for rearing. If implemented, these laws can help ban poultry's confinement to battery cages or pigs to gestation crates. The road to the humane treatment of farm animals, if possible, is long and filled with unreasonable hurdles blanketed by unfair laws and practices.

The Reality of Factory Farms

Overlook Animal Welfare

Intensive animal farming is profit-oriented and overlooks the need for animal welfare. In this process, animals are nothing more than mere commodities raised for earning a profit. This becomes a significant hurdle, especially when the livestock contracts any illnesses. Instead of using resources to speed up the recovery and raise healthier animals, the profitable option is to send them to slaughter. It is easier to start over than aiding their recovery. Pneumonia is an extremely common health problem across different species.

As mentioned in the previous chapter, the illnesses these animals develop during farming practices are harmful to humans too. It all started with animal-borne diseases from the spread of the avian flu to the latest COVID-19 pandemic.

Restricted Movements

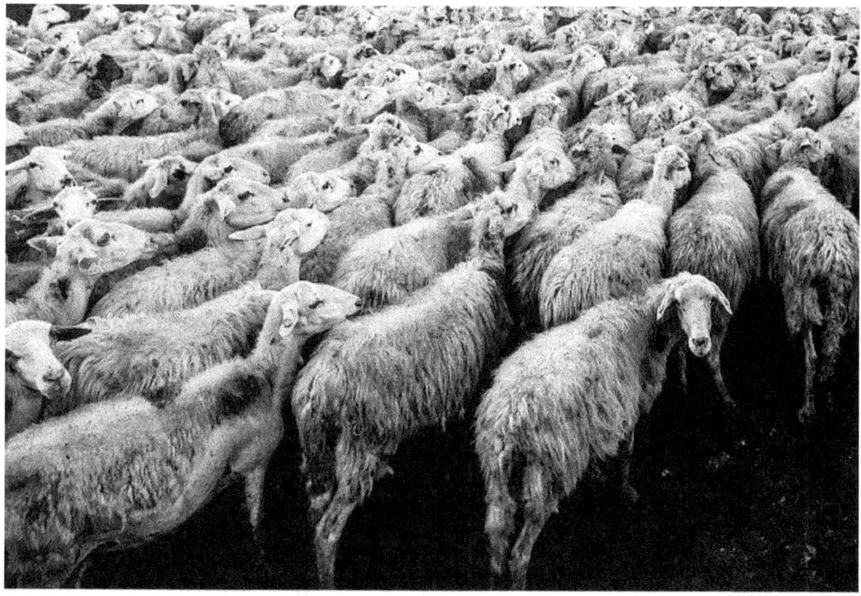

More food and less space seem to be the motto of intensive animal farming methods. It helps produce great results when compared with conventional family-based operations. The lack of space forces these animals into overcrowded environments that essentially restrict their movement. Apart from the ethical considerations, movement restriction also harms their overall health. Trimming the tips of wings or parts of hooves are common practices in factory farming as these help to restrict movement. In the end, all this impacts the quality of food thus produced.

Disadvantages of Mesh Floors

In intensive farming methods, managing animal waste is a critical issue. The simplest and most efficient way to do this is by using mesh floors, making it easier to pass urine and feces. It optimizes the cleaning process, but the mesh floors can harm their feet. This is also believed to be a reason for the increased fat content in the animal proteins available today.

Genetic Manipulation

Factory farming and genetic engineering go hand-in-hand. Genetic engineering helps develop superior species that provide better results. It, in turn, helps increase the overall profitability without increasing the costs involved. It essentially is a process that makes these animals more useful to humans. There are different animal welfare issues caused due to selective breeding. Chickens are genetically engineered to lay more than 300 eggs annually, while sows are bred to birth large litters. These numbers are impossible if these animals were left in their natural habitat. It increases profitability, but seriously harms the health of the animals. From calcium deficiencies to hormonal imbalances and reduced immunity, these animals endure a lot of suffering. When animals are modified to grow faster or produce more milk, we are merely increasing the suffering endured by these overworked animals living in pathetic conditions.

Intensive farming prioritizes results and justifies the means if they provide the desired results. Therefore, it isn't unusual for most facilities to crossbreed different species for generating desirable growth behaviors. Artificial stimulants promote their growth and increase their weight as required. Unsurprisingly, the birth to processing timeframe is reduced by more than 50%. This is not just unnatural, but undesirable too. Most animals grow to unnatural proportions. Evolution is natural and desirable. However, human intervention has wreaked havoc and thoroughly disrupted this natural process. Gene editing and genetic engineering have reduced the food per day requirement for farm breeding. A combination of these factors harms the health of these animals while increasing the profit margins.

Unnatural Changes

After going through the molting process, hens usually lay one egg every day. If the chickens are forced into darkness for eight hours, devoid of water and food, they can lay a second egg. Even if one out of every ten hens die due to this process, the overall production levels increase and help maximize the profitability of such farms. These days, cattle are artificially inseminated to trigger earlier production of milk. Cows are also maintained in a constant state of pregnancy to optimize milk production. Once the dairy production stops, the cattle are sent to slaughterhouses, and the same process starts again.

Family Separation

With intensive farming methods, family separation is quite common. Piglets are separated from sows within two weeks, which ends the weaning process. It also prepares the sow for quick and successive pregnancies. Dairy facilities separate the calves from their mothers' days after birth to increase milk production. Lambs and calves are also sent to the slaughter for food supply. The average lifespan of a dairy cow these days is only five years, instead of 20 years like it is supposed to be because of all the intensive farming techniques. It increases the production of dairy but harms their health.

Lack of Vet Care

Veterinary care is not only expensive, but it disrupts the production cycle, too. Taking care of sick animals is expensive, and therefore, most factories prefer slaughtering animals when they get sick. These animals become a part of the regular food supply. Factory farming depends on the extensive use of antibiotics to prevent any illnesses. It might help reduce the overall cost of these animals' maintenance, but it ultimately leads to their demise or ends up contaminating the food supply.

No Natural Behaviors

All the animals that live in a factory farm are prevented from exhibiting their natural behaviors. The main reason for this is the lack of space, and secondly, genetic engineering. In an ideal environment, swine and hogs often spend their days idling away in the sun. Likewise, cows prefer grazing in pastures all day long. However, on a factory farm, none of this is possible, and they are all confined to closed indoor environments. These animals never get a chance to be the animals they were born to be.

Chilling Statistics

For thousands of years, humans have been farming animals, but things changed drastically over the last 100 years. The animals are housed, fed, handled, and their production processes have all been designed to meet the increasing demand for animal foods. This increase in factory farming means several billions of animals have and are still enduring lives that are downright cruel and inhumane. A life where they are restricted to tiny cages, unable to extend their limbs or flap their wings, denied an opportunity to breathe fresh air, and kept from living like they were supposed to.

Can you imagine being cramped up in a room for as long as you live? Well, this is what battery chickens experience. Chickens raised on factory farms live in extremely compact cages with an A4 floor size. There is barely any room for these chickens to turn around, let alone flap their wings. The mesh flooring used to ease the cleaning process is extremely uncomfortable and the birds end up standing on it for most of their lives before being sent to their death. Excessive pain, injuries, and discomfort are common, but the normal reality in factory farms.

The cramped up and messy conditions of a factory farm increase the exposure of different animals to various illnesses. According to a study conducted by Horrigan et al., (2002), approximately 60-65% of pigs test positive for pneumonia-like lesions on the lungs. It is believed this is caused due to massive amounts of ammonia and harmful gases released by the humongous quantities of manure these animals produce and come in contact with daily. Most of the pigs that enter the United States slaughterhouses have pneumonia!

Despite knowing that animals can live, breathe, and feel, they aren't treated as sentient beings. Instead, their sole purpose is to fulfill human needs by meeting a cruel end. We all need to accept these hard truths to understand how the food we eat is sourced fully. Let us look at some chilling statistics which showcase the harsh reality of factory farming animals.

Chickens

According to a white paper titled, "Selective Breeding In The Chicken Industry: The Case For Slower Growth," published by the ASPCA (American Society for the prevention of cruelty to animals) suggests around 9 billion chickens are killed annually for meat. In comparison, 300 million chickens are reared for laying eggs. Unfortunately, all poultry such as ducks, geese, meat, chicken, egg-laying hens, turkeys, and so on aren't covered under any existing federal laws. Given their sheer numbers and the cruel lives they are forced to live, it is high time for some positive change. Another common problem in the intensive factory farming industry is selective breeding and utilization of weight gaining drugs. When animals are fed these drugs, their growth rate is drastically altered.

For instance, a normal chicken takes about 90 days to reach the desired weight for slaughter. These days, chickens are slaughtered within 35 days. Also, these animals can attain the desired weight, even when there is a drastic reduction in their feed. In the 1950s, to produce one pound of meat, the animals had to be fed 3 pounds of feed. These days, the average feed has come down to 1.7 pounds.

Windowless sheds with several rows of battery cages are the housing unit for approximately 300,000,000 egg-laying hens in the United States alone. Each cage, the size of a file drawer, houses around ten hens within its wiry and severely uncomfortable structure. When these birds are packed in such horrible conditions, they develop abnormal behaviors and indulge in cannibalism. To prevent such behaviors, a sensitive portion of their beak is often burnt or cut off. Another barbaric truth is gender discrimination.

Only female chickens can lay eggs, and about half of the chicks hatched in the poultry industry turn out to be male. A male chick takes a long time to grow and is often lanky, unlike the meat chickens. So, what happens to these chicks? Since rearing them is an expensive process, they are often slaughtered right at birth. If the egg production rate of a hen decreases due to age or any other factor, it is killed or sent to slaughter. Another cruel yet widely prevalent tactic is to starve the bird for approximately 14 days to send its body into a final molt. In 1999, the system of battery cages was banned by the European Union. However, this ban allowed a slow 12-year phase-out period. This merely goes on to show the willingness of humans to turn a blind eye towards the suffering of animals for their gains.

Turkeys

In the United States alone, 240 million turkeys are raised for their meat. As with chickens, these birds are bred in small and compact cages with hardly any room for movement. Did you know that the modern turkey doesn't resemble its wild ancestors? The disproportionately breast-heavy birds we see today are the result of genetic selection based on the consumer's widespread demand for breast meat. These birds are grown quite quickly, and their disproportionate body structure results in physical ailments such as the inability to breathe or walk properly. They are also subjected to year-round artificial insemination, which further ruins their health. By nature's design, turkeys are meant to reproduce only once annually. However, these numbers cannot sustain the demand for turkey meat and resulted in human intervention via genetic alterations. This is also why the average weight of a turkey increased from 13 to 30 pounds between 1930 and 2017.

Cattle

There are no standardized or uniform laws and regulations about rearing cattle. Practices differ from one industry to another. Cattle are raised for beef, dairy, and veal. Unlike other factory-farmed animals, the cattle raised for their beef, are the only farm animals that are mostly raised outdoors. However, once the animals are between the ages of six months and a year, they are sent to live in feedlots cramped with hundreds or even thousands of other cattle until slaughter.

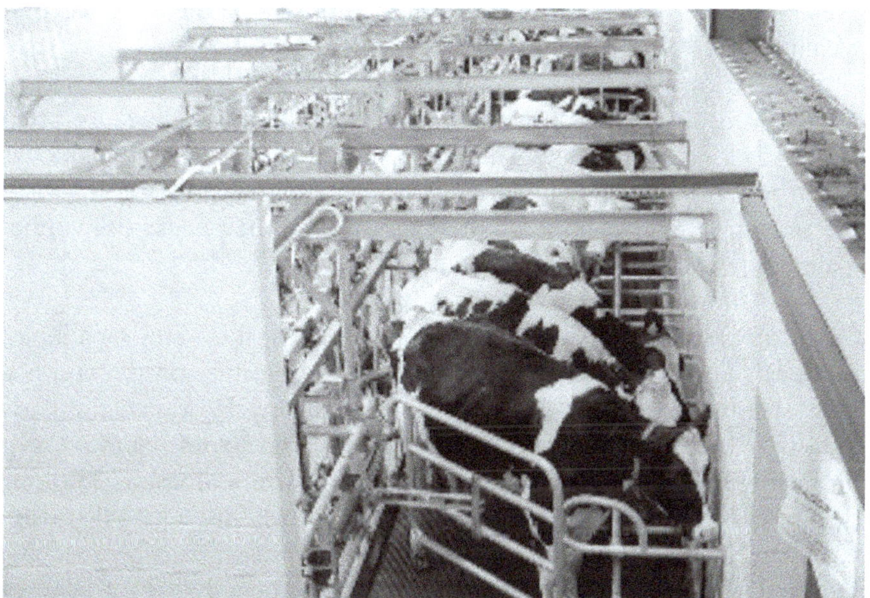

These animals are often forced to live without proper shelter or even sufficient vegetated pastures. It, in turn, harms their health and causes severe digestive distress. Corn and a combination of other grains are used as feed. These foods are not what cattle are used to eating. They are designed to live outdoors and graze hay. Instead, they are forced to live in congested spaces that restrict their movement. The stress of living in such conditions combined with a horrible diet and indoor conditions severely harms their health. Rather distressing practices such as branding and castration are the norm and cause extreme pain and discomfort to these animals. They are often forced to endure the trauma of transport when moved across state lines.

According to the study "The Psychology of Cows" (2017), cattle are considered social animals displaying and understanding the concepts of herd hierarchies. They are also capable of forming strong bonds with their young ones. There were instances when a cow kept calling out to her calf when separated. These animals also respond to those around them and how they are handled. A corn and soy diet, such as the one fed to most beef cattle, is not their ideal form of sustenance. Forced to live on an unnatural diet causes severe gastric distress and illnesses such as ulcers. Most cattle are "grass-fed" because they start their young lives by feeding on grass. They eat grass until sent to the feedlots, after which they are slaughtered.

Cattle are used not just for beef, but dairy too. Dairy cows are often housed indoors, while others might be allowed to live in dirty paddocks or left in outdoor concrete structures. They are never allowed to roam free and are often left tethered by chains around their necks or by other materials known as tie stalls.

Cows are mammals. So, like human females, they are capable of producing milk only after giving birth. In a way, milk production is a side-effect of pregnancy and subsequent delivery. However, the dairy industry thrives on this milk produced. The cows cannot keep producing milk after nursing and weaning their little ones. To prolong this process of producing milk, cows are artificially inseminated at dairy farms at least once a year. A cow's gestation period usually lasts nine months, and therefore, most dairy cows live their lives in a state of perpetual pregnancy. This results in the unnaturally high amount of milk they produce.

On the downside, it causes a painful bacterial infection known as mastitis, which harms the cow's udders. They not only have to live with this discomfort, but also their pain doesn't end here. Calves don't even get a chance to nurse young ones after pregnancy. If the young calf consumes all this milk, it reduces dairy production. Therefore, calves are often removed from their mother on the day of the birth itself. This is traumatic for the mother and the calf too. If it is a female calf, she would be used as the next-generation dairy cows while the male would be raised for veal.

Once again, as with any other species that's factory-farmed, even these cows exhibit unnatural behaviors due to their living conditions and physical health. The answer to these problems is another barbaric method of removing the cow's horns and cutting up two-thirds of their tails without administering any painkillers. Somehow, the animal industry has come up with a cruel answer to a cruel human-made problem. The cattle industry is interconnected even if the dairy operations are held separately from beef cattle. Once the dairy cows stop producing milk, the milk production has gone down, or they cannot produce milk, either due to age or illness, they are sent to slaughterhouses. These cows make a quick shift and go from a milk-producing machine to being slaughtered for beef.

The genetically engineered dairy cows used in the dairy industry can produce anywhere between 50-100 pounds of milk daily. This figure is ten times higher than what it was in the last couple of decades. Selective breeding, administering growth hormones, and following an unnatural diet are some of the reasons for this startling increase. More than 9 million cows are used for producing milk per year in the US alone. A majority of downed animals, the ones who can no longer stand or walk, are dairy cows. The natural lifespan of a healthy cow is anywhere between 20-25 years. The aggressively bred dairy cows are forced to produce as much quality milk as they possibly can, which is considered to be for only three lactation cycles. A majority of these cows end up in the slaughterhouse before they are even five years old. Sending these cows to an early slaughter is a cheaper and more profitable option than tending to them.

Veal

Veal is an incredibly popular and tender meat. It is also quite expensive. Do you know where veal comes from? A lot of people wrongly believe veal is the same as beef. No, veal comes from young cattle raised solely for early slaughter. Veal calves are usually the young cattle birthed by dairy cows. Since the female calves are used as next-generation dairy cows, the male calves left over. These calves don't have much use for the dairy or meat industry in general. Therefore, they are sent to the slaughterhouse and sold as expensive meats later. Traditionally, veal is pale meat, and this color was obtained by restricting the diet and movement of these calves. This is also the reason why veal is one of the most tender meats available. The muscles in their bodies are not yet fully developed, making them pliant and tender. Usually, once the calves are six-weeks-old, they are all housed together in crowded groups with insufficient movement space, denied any exercise and solid food, which goes against their early instinct to suckle. If the dairy industry didn't exist, the veal industry would not survive. After all, these calves are obtained from dairy calves. By sending the male calves to an early slaughter, it is one less mouth to feed for this gigantic and cruel meat industry with deep pockets.

Pigs

Every year, approximately 120,000,000 pigs are raised for food in the United States alone. Most of them are reared in tiny pens or barren crates at factory-like operations without any exposure to the natural surroundings. Pigs have a natural urge to root and often spend a lot of their time sunning or rooting in mud. They are deprived of their natural habitat due to factory farming and are instead forced to live on slatted floors. The continuous exposure to manure and lack of proper hygiene and sanitation, increases the levels of ammonia.

As mentioned earlier, excess and prolonged exposure to ammonia increases the chances of pneumonia. Pigs are naturally intelligent and curious beings. When restricted to such congested and barren living conditions, they become frustrated. A common unnatural behavior showcased by pigs in such conditions is fighting. To prevent this, industries have started chipping or cutting off a small portion of their teeth and nails to prevent biting. All of this is done without administering any anesthetics.

Sows are confined to gestational crates for the entirety of their reproductive life cycle. The crates they are accommodated in are extremely congested and barely allow any space for movement. Intensive farming practices include artificial insemination of these sows who are later transferred from their restrictive gestational crates to farrowing crates before delivery. Sows stay in these crates for nursing their young ones for two weeks, after which they are immediately transferred to gestational crates for artificial insemination. This process goes on until the sow is no longer fit to reproduce or dies in this process. If the sow is no longer useful, it is immediately sent for slaughter.

Seafood

A lot of people wrongly believe fish and other aquatic animals are incapable of feeling any pain whatsoever. They might not be able to express their pain the way land animals can do, but they are also sentient beings. Fish and other aquatic vertebrates can experience fear and suffering. One of the quickest growing areas of food production in the world today is aquaculture. In aquaculture, a specific species of fish and other aquatic species are farmed solely for supplying food. Most of the popular species of fish such as trout, salmon, tuna, cod, and halibut are not fish from the oceans but are farmed artificially. Unnaturally created habitats, specially designed to raise specific aquatic species for food production is becoming a serious global problem.

The animals that live on land-based animal farms exist in overcrowded conditions. Likewise, even the fish in these units are overcrowded. Industrial fisheries are breeding grounds for disease-causing pathogens, which increases the need for these fisheries to rely on antibiotics. These antibiotics leave residues that enter the human food chain. Growing fish in unnatural conditions harms their wellbeing and is a cause of concern. Stunning fish before slaughter would sound like a humane option. Unfortunately, this isn't the reality. Instead, these species are allowed to slowly and painfully die by bleeding out, using blunt force trauma, freezing, or even suffocation in some cases. Fish grown in industrial fisheries are often carnivores. These fish depend on other smaller fish for sustenance. To produce a pound of farmed salmon or any other variety of predatory fish, up to four pounds of feeder fish is needed.

Since intensive factory farming is all about economies of scale, taking care of the animals is never a priority. Not just a priority, but it is a simple aspect that is always overlooked. The fact that all these animals with life and feelings are bred and grown in inhumane conditions is never even considered in this industry. Even if it sounds brutal and paints a vivid, horrible picture, it is a wake-up call. Unless you understand these statistics, you can't fully understand the cruel treatment these innocent animals are bred to endure. After a miserable existence, the only relief they get is death.

Impact of Factory Farming

Intensive factory farming is not only inhumane and barbaric to the animals, but it also isn't good for everyone else involved. From the environment to the ultimate consumers, everything is sustaining damage because of these unnatural practices.

Human Health

In the previous chapters, you were introduced to the different harmful effects of meat and other animal foods on human health. Poorly maintained farms become breeding grounds for harmful bacteria such as E. Coli, salmonella, and other disease-inducing pathogens. All these pathogens are passed on to humans via eggs, meat, dairy products, and even human-to-human contact. Since animals are living in such unsanitary habitats, they are pumped with antibiotics. Excessive and improper use of such harmful antibiotics enters the human food chain leading to the development of lethal and drug-resistant pathogens, which can spread amongst humans and animals. Be it swine flu or the coronavirus; these are startling examples of the diseases spread via animal foods.

The Environment

Intensive factory farming is wreaking havoc on our environment. Precious resources such as land, water, and air are polluted from the waste produced by factory farms. It's not just the neighboring communities that suffer; it compromises the global environment and leads to excessive pollution. These pollutants don't go away and once again harm humans and every living being on earth. Finite resources such as fossil fuels and water are consumed in humongous quantities by these facilities. These resources are depleting, but the carbon footprint is steadily increasing due to the harmful emissions. It is believed industrial animal agriculture produces more than 400 different types of toxic gases. More greenhouse gases are generated due to these practices than the summation of the total global transport.

Workers

All the low-level individuals engaged in these processes, such as farmworkers and laborers, are among the lowest-paid employees within the United States. The pay they get is highly disproportionate to the risks they face. It is saddening to note that the federal labor laws do not apply to these workers. They miss out on laws that provide essential protections such as their right to organize, or the right to overtime. Prolonged exposure to a hazardous environment and other disease-causing pathogens are some of the common risks these workers face.

The Toll on Rural Communities

The environmental pollution caused by these practices makes it difficult for rural communities to enjoy a good quality of life. Contaminated drinking water, polluted air, and the lack of outdoor spaces are only some of the problems those residing near such establishments face. For instance, the study conducted by (Nicole et al., 2013) shows the adverse effects of intensive factory farming on rural areas' health and environment.

Apart from the rural communities, it's wiping out the concept of independent family farms in the United States. From 5.6 million farms in 1950, the number reduced to 2 million farms in 2017. However, the number of animals raised on these farms increased from 100 million to 9.32 billion. This shows how the corporatization of industrial agriculture is slowly but certainly killing the system of independent family farms and affecting the livelihoods of tens of thousands.

Are Pasture-Raised and Grass-Fed Options More Humane?

What is the first thing that pops into your head when you think about pasture-raised and grass-fed meats and animal products? You perhaps imagine a charming and picturesque farm with vast pastures speckled with freely roaming animals. This is a pleasant thought, isn't it? Well, the reality is quite different. There is an ever-increasing demand for pasture-raised and grass-fed options these days. Perhaps a lot of people look for these options because they believe it to be more humane. Another reason for this increasing popularity is the belief these options are healthier and more nutritious when compared with factory-farmed animal foods. If you had an opportunity to visit such a farm, you would start believing or even wishing that all animals were raised like this. This is an idealistic figment of your imagination and not reality.

These days, consumers are certainly going out of their way to purchase cage-free or pasture-raised eggs and meat from the local farmer's markets. Locally sourced produce seems to be a buzzword. Some studies show that about 75% of adults in the US believe that animal foods they consume are sourced humanely. However, according to the estimates gathered by Sentience Institute suggest more than 99% of the animals farmed within the United States live on concentrated animal feeding operations or factory farms. If you look at these numbers globally, it will mean over 90% of the animal foods available in the market are not sourced humanely.

In fact, this raises another question about what the term 'humane' actually means. How humane is it to use animals as our food source and not treat them as living beings? For instance, what do cage-free eggs mean? It essentially means the birds are not confined to cages and are allowed to roam in the open. Most poultry is not raised in cages, and they are bred in tightly packed sheds. Technically, the eggs derived from such a source can be termed "cage-free." The space available per bird, however, will still stay the same.

Even if animals aren't restricted to cages, it isn't always a pretty picture. Just because these animals are roaming in the open, doesn't mean they are happy and healthy. There are several instances where the animals living in such a stressful environment often die from the high-density confinement. The air quality is often worse on cage-free farms because all the animals are walking around, kicking up dust, and leaving feces behind. This certainly doesn't seem like a safe source to obtain your nourishment from. When animals are raised on pastures, some of these problems can be avoided to a certain degree. However, new issues tend to crop up. The most common issues associated with pasture-based flocks are predation and the threat of infections from other wild animals.

Believe it or not, grass-fed cow farming is worse when compared to grain-fed cow farming. The production of methane, a leading greenhouse gas, is twice as high as those generated from grain-fed cow farming. More precious resources, such as land, water, and fossil fuels, are required to produce grass-fed beef. Before you purchase any grass-fed or pasture-raised meats, remember it increases your share carbon emission or your carbon footprint. There certainly are some farms that prioritize the animal's welfare. However, ending their life is indeed a terrible experience.

Ethical animal farming is nothing more than a mirage. It's an idea that's highly unlikely, and it's merely a way to assuage your guilt of consuming animal foods. Over the years, there have been undercover investigations and scientific reports that showcase animal farming's environmental effect. However, most of us have decided to turn a blind eye towards the data right in front of us. As mentioned in the earlier section, animal farming does no good whatsoever. When it comes to animal suffering or environmental damage, there is only one choice—end animal farming. Irrespective of whether the animals are caged or allowed to roam freely, in the end, they are all slaughtered for human consumption.

There is possibly no way in which such rampant slaughter can be justified. Ethical farming is not a reality. In fact, the animals might be in a worse situation than they would be in a factory. Several animals die from infections, cancer, and other health problems. Artificial breeding sends their reproductive systems into overdrive. Even if you keep aside the ethical drawbacks, let us consider the numbers. A dozen eggs from an ethical animal farm costs $6 and upwards. Most of the population would not be willing to shell out such big bucks for a mere dozen eggs. The numbers sound unpleasant, but this is the reality.

The need of the hour is to pass and enforce extensive regulations and prioritize animal welfare. Even if the theory of humane animal farming can be turned into a reality, it certainly is not feasible fiscally at this time. Subjecting animals to an existence riddled with cruelty and endless pain because of low prices and high profits is not an ethical solution. Instead, it's time to take a giant step forward and abolish the idea of animal farming altogether. Plant-based diets are not only healthy and nutritious, but they are environmentally and ethically merciful too.

Chapter Four:

Climate Change and Animal Farming

Climate change is one of the harsh realities of the modern world. In the past, the world focused on how to prevent or reduce the emission of greenhouse gases and other chemicals, but it is more prudent for people to now focus on agriculture, especially animal agriculture or farming. Steven Chu, a Noble prizewinner and the former Energy Secretary, looked at various factories and industries, and noted that the meat and dairy industry pollutes the environment more than any other industry.

Chu stated that dairy cows and cattle emit more greenhouse gases when compared to the European Union and the United States. Chu is currently the President of the American Association for the Advancement of Science, so his opinion is one to listen to!

During his research, Chu looked at the greenhouse gas emission from dairy and meat industry, and compared these emissions with the emissions of land-use changes, such as soil disruption and deforestation and various agricultural practices, like the use of fertilizers. He looked at the resulting weights, and measured the potency and lifetime of these emissions. His results showed that the emissions from agriculture were higher when compared to the emissions from other sectors and industries, like energy.

Chu also talked about industrial agriculture and its unnatural effects. He termed the produce as oversexed corn, and also found that this corn was used to feed pigs (so they gained 280 pounds in a few months) and turkeys (so they have juicier breasts and could not mate). Farmers used many resources to make giant kernels. He stated that our planet is now dominated by modified and artificially inseminated animals who were only raised and slaughtered to feed the growing population.

According to the survey, "The biomass distribution on Earth (2018)," people and the animals they eat contribute to at least 96% of the carbon mass in the world. Chu further stated that only 4% of the carbon mass in the world is because of rats, mice, lions and buffalos.

It is important to understand that Chu is probably one of the many experts who stated that animal agriculture contributes to climate change. Chu believes the easiest way to overcome this climate change is through biotechnology. He mentioned that they could use a symbiotic fertilizer to develop fake or faux meat. That said, it does not make sense to do this since there will be more factories set up to develop this meat. Therefore, the simplest solution to this scary problem would be to shift to a plant-based diet.

Why Should You Follow a Plant-Based Diet?

Many dieticians and nutritionists believe people should switch to a plant-based diet. It is important for us to be aware of what we eat, so we do not add to the carbon footprint on the planet. A plant-based diet is based on grains, fruits, and vegetables that reduce the land and water used for production. This diet also reduces soil erosion, deforestation, and pollution.

International Peace is an Added Bonus

The Office of the Director of National Intelligence released a recent report that highlights the threat of water shortages across the nation. This report also found that the pressure on freshwater resources, along with increased flooding and poor water quality, might lead to negative effects on various international initiatives. This report was released in March 2020 and concluded by saying that it would be prudent for people to change their diets to reduce the water used for animal agriculture and farming. This is the only way to reduce water scarcity.

This report does not go into too much detail about the changes that must be made since livestock consumes a lot of water. Therefore, when the factory farming industry scales back on the water used to cultivate crops to feed animals, it can prevent water shortages across the globe.

You Should Follow a Plant-Based Diet According to the UN

The United Nations stated that humans should move from a meat-based or animal-product based diet to a plant-based diet. There are over 7 billion people on the planet now, and the number is predicted to increase by another 2 billion by the year 2050. The UN states that most of the water that people consume is often used only to produce food. The UN also has tried to educate people about the repercussions of a meat-based diet. It tells people how the production of meat uses more than a hundred times the water used to cultivate plant-based foods for people. For instance, it takes 15,000 liters of water to produce only one pound of beef, while it takes only 1,500 liters of water to produce one pound of wheat. These statistics show that on an average, 150 grams of meat uses more than 2,025 liters of water when compared to the 69 liters of water used to produce the same quantity of wheat. These statistics paint an accurate picture of the harsh realities of the meat industry.

Depletion of Water Availability and Quality

The United States uses more than half the water present in the country for animal harvesting and agriculture. One of the best examples of this overexploitation is of the Aquifer that stretches between Texas and the Dakotas. The people around this region use this aquifer for irrigation, and over 60% of the livestock is raised in this region. This region also produces large quantities of corn, and most of it is used to feed the livestock raised in the area.

Since corn needs a lot of water during its growth, it was impossible to grow it in the Great Plains without taking water from the aquifer. The Ogallala aquifer was found in 1911, and the water is depleting at a rapid rate. Experts believe that the water may deplete completely in another 20 years. Animal farms not only exhaust water resources, but they also pollute various water bodies.

Farmed animals produce more than 100 times more manure when compared to people in the area, and since there is absolutely no way to treat animal waste, the toxins and other particles in the waste pollutes nearby waterways. For example, a lagoon in North Carolina that was eight acres long burst in 1995. Due to this spill, over 25 million gallons of toxins and chemicals from animal waste was pumped into The New River. This closed off 364,000 acres of wetlands near the coast and killed over 10 million fish. People hoped that this was only an isolated incident, but there were more pollution incidents, including 1000 spills, between the years 1995 and 1998. This resulted in the death of over 13 million fish.

Animal waste also releases both nitrous oxide and methane, and these gases are the major contributors of climate change and environmental damage. The potency of methane is 23 times more than carbon dioxide, and that of nitrous oxide is 300 times greater than both carbon dioxide and methane. Global warming is linked to various natural disasters, including flooding and water logging across the world. The livestock industry is responsible for numerous problems, and the National Intelligence agency noted that this industry is responsible for the pollution of water supplies and overuse of nonrenewable water sources thereby leading to global warming.

Even if we overlook the unethical practices of rampant animal cruelty in the meat industry, it is impossible to ignore its environmental implications.

Governments Now Motivate People to Follow Plant-based Diets

Members of international and local governments and policymakers in the United Nations and other countries and cities have taken notice of the benefits of the plant-based diet on the environment. Tulsi Gabbard, a Councilwoman from Honolulu City, conducted a rally recently to help people understand various sustainable solutions and their need to implement those solutions to support the environment. She believed that if families made at least one change in their lives, it could have a ripple effect throughout the community. She also mentioned when one person makes a change in the family, it becomes easier to motivate others in the family and the community, and this would help the city overcome its health and environmental problems. She asked people to switch from a meat-based diet to a plant-based diet, where they only consumed fruit, vegetables, whole grains, and plants.

It is important to understand that raising animals for food leads to water pollution, air pollution, overuse of resources and soil erosion, all of which are wreaking havoc on Earth. The most important thing people should do to improve the environment and their health is to switch to a vegetarian diet—now!

How Can You Contribute?

We can all make a difference if we come together. The easiest and most practical option to counter these challenges is by following a plant-based diet or at least reducing your intake of animal products. This paves way to a greener and brighter future on Earth. Let us look at some ways you can contribute to protecting the Earth.

Reduce Your Carbon Footprint

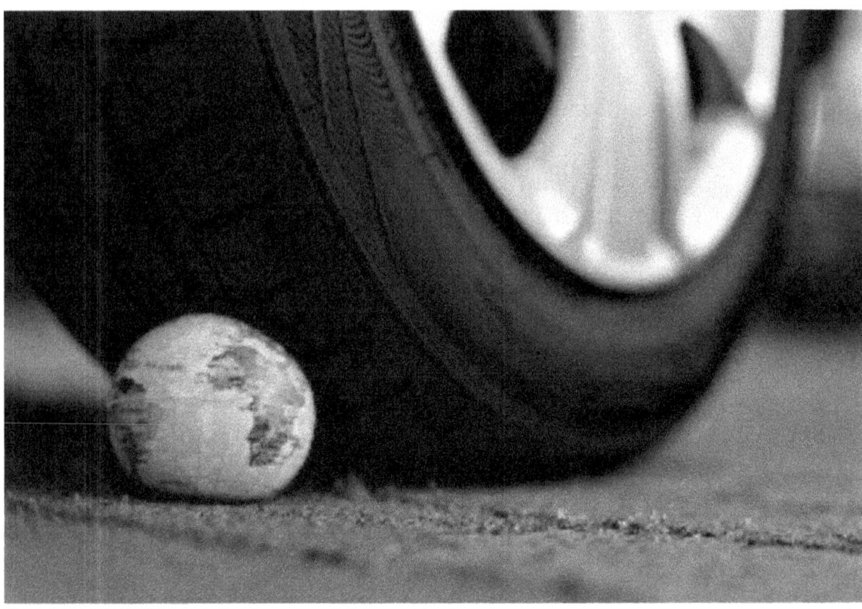

From the information above, we have seen that animal agriculture leads to global warming and deforestation. According to the Food and Agriculture Organization (FAO), a United Nations department, estimated that more than 14.5% of the global emissions of greenhouse gases is due to the production of livestock. Some organizations believe that the emissions could be greater than 50%.

It is also important to understand that the manure produced is not just disgusting, but it also contributes to more than 37% of the global greenhouse gas emissions. Manure produces large quantities of methane, and since most factories do not manage manure well, the gas warms the earth faster than carbon dioxide. If you add the fuel used to transport and grow feed for livestock, the carbon footprint gets even higher.

Conserve Water

Do you know how many gallons of water are used to produce a carton of milk? The Water Footprint Network says factories take more than 1000 gallons of water to produce just one liter of milk. If you are earth-conscious, then this statistic should convince you to avoid animal products. A survey conducted by the Pew Commission on Industrial Farm Animal Production concluded that more than 87% of the water used in the US is for Agriculture. If you add the amount of water it takes to produce meat when compared to the amount it takes to produce one pound of grains, it must be making a pretty good case for you to reduce your intake of animal protein.

Save Plant and Animal Habitats

Did you know that we currently use more than a third of land that could be used to grow crops, instead it is used for animal agriculture? We use that land to feed chicken, cattle, and pigs. It is for this reason why animal agriculture is one of the biggest contributors to desertification and deforestation. The former is the phenomenon where natural vegetation is destroyed due to livestock grazing, which leads to soil erosion. These phenomena lead to the extinction of numerous species, such as sloths, orangutans, and red pandas. Many animals in the US are also affected due to animal agriculture, and it is estimated that at least 33% and 14% of endangered or threatened plants and animals, respectively, are affected by livestock grazing.

Dead Zones

Animal husbandry or agriculture is one of the main reasons for water pollution, and also increases the dead zones in oceans. The waste from most factory farms are stored and applied as fertilizer to crops around the factory. This waste is untreated, and thus numerous toxins are released into the earth. Since the soil cannot absorb such large quantities of toxins from the manure, they move to the groundwater and finally into oceans and rivers. This destroys various ecosystems in the ocean. A great example of such a dead zone is the 8,500 square foot region in the Mississippi River that became a dead zone since the water was polluted with animal and farm waste from the Midwest. This dead zone made it impossible for marine life to survive.

Clean Air

Do you remember the tons of manure we talked about earlier? Well, that mass also produces ammonia, which is one of the most potent forms of nitrogen. It causes algae blooms, increases smog in the air, and kills fish. Additionally, the air that surrounds factory farms contains various greenhouse gases, including methane and carbon dioxide, and other gases and particulate matter that pollutes the environment. When you switch to a plant-based diet, you do not depend on the food produced in these factories, and therefore reduce the emissions of these gases one plant-based meal at a time.

Chapter Five:

Ending World Hunger by Going Plant-Based

People have been talking about how important it is for everybody to follow a vegetarian or vegan diet to end world hunger. If nutritious grains were used to feed humans instead of animals, world hunger would eventually disappear. The demand for crops is increasing worldwide due to the increase in global population, the demand is also changing in regards to dietary preferences and a leaning toward production of biofuel.

It is a substantial challenge to meet these growing demands, which eventually taxes the capability of the food system. This growing demand requires governments to increase their crop production. It would, in turn, increase the availability of food by 70%. This increase in food availability can feed at least 4 billion people.

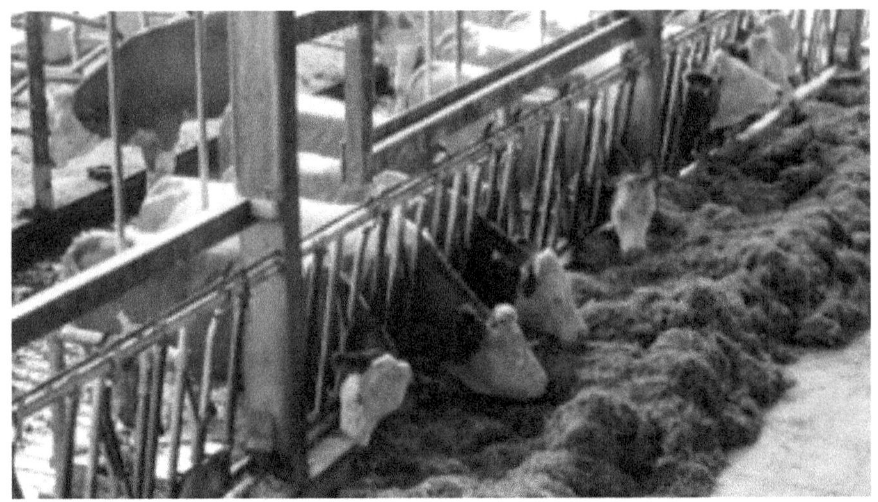

A team of researchers from the Environment department at the University of Minnesota found that farmed animals eat more than 36 percent of calories from crops. The study conducted by Cassidy et al., (2013) states that people only eat 12% of those calories when they eat meat, which is a two-third drop in the number of calories consumed. If people were fed those grains instead, they could have consumed that many more calories. This team also found that when people grow crops only for human consumption, the available

food increases by 70% and this can feed at least 4 billion people. This increase is more than enough to feed the growing population. Yes, it is as simple as it sounds. World hunger is a serious problem and we can all end it by opting for sustainable diets!

This same study also says that it takes at least 13 pounds of grain to produce one pound of meat, and if these grains were used to feed people instead of animals, there will be enough to feed everybody who does not have much to eat. Malnutrition affects more than 800 million people across the globe, and this issue is the cause of death of more than 3.1 million children below the age of five each year.

Research shows that pigs, chickens and cows raised for food often suffer every day, and they endure a terrifying and painful death. When you drink their milk, eat their eggs or flesh, you suffer too, since animal products are linked to almost everything from diabetes to heart disease. These products can also increase the risk of obesity and cancer. When you feed these animals lots of crops, including grains, you take all this food out of children's mouths.

The best thing you should do for your own health, the planet, and animals is to follow a plant-based diet. In light of the study mentioned above, it can be seen that a plant-based diet is probably the only way to prevent further damage to the planet. This same study also shows that dairy products, meat, and eggs damage the body.

Numerous studies show there is a significant association between pandemic diseases, such as obesity and diabetes, and diet. According to a study on the implications of the western diet on climate change conducted by (Vega et al., 2018), your current eating habits not only affect your health, but also affect agricultural production and the environment. Earlier studies in this field show that there was a relationship between eating habits and each of the topics mentioned earlier. This study analyzes the link or relationship between environmental data, health, and agricultural production. The research team used a global database to collect this data, and found that the Western diet negatively impacts all three since it is dominated by refined sugars, flour, processed food, and fats. They found that an increased consumption and production of refined grains and sugars over the last few years is related to negative outcomes, such as obesity and diabetes.

It was also noted that our eating habits clear large forest areas and produce huge quantities of GHGe. In this study, the team looked at three databases between the years 1975 and 2015:

- Health data obtained from the 2018 WHO database
- Environmental data obtained from the 2018 FAOSTAT database

- Agricultural data obtained from the 2018 FAOSTAT database

The team conducted numerous analyses using the data from these databases, and compared the results with the global population growth. They included the global population growth in their analysis to eliminate that the correlations derived from the analysis are associated with only the demographic behavior.

Did you know that the consumption of sugar tripled in the last 50 years, and the production of oils and sweeteners has largely increased? It is important to note that these are the main ingredients of this diet. For instance, the production of sugarcane has increased by 294% in the last five decades, and so has the production of corn.

A lot of energy goes into the production of these items, which leads to the emission of CH4 and CO2. In the last few years, the emission of these gases has doubled, but the use of land for agricultural use has decreased globally. Several areas in the world now suffer from diet-related crises combined with food security and environmental issues. These health crises are characterized by overweight, obesity, malnutrition, and some metabolic and nutrient-related disorders, such as hypertension, cancer, Type 2 Diabetes and cardiovascular disease. The percentage of childhood obesity has increased from 1% to 7%, and so has diabetes. These issues have both environmental and economic consequences, and the health system has collapsed in numerous countries since they do not have the resources to cater to their citizens' lifestyle.

Research teams from both Oxford University and the University of Minnesota looked at the effect of 15 common foods in the Western diet, and connected their effect on human health. They also examined the correlation between the 15 foods and environmental damage. They also associated these foods with potential health outcomes and some aspects of environmental degradation.

The team of researchers also looked at various plant-based items, such as potatoes, nuts, seeds, legumes, fruit, vegetables, whole grain cereals and refined grains and animal-foods, such as processed and raw red meat, fish, eggs, dairy products and chicken. They used the data from the global databases mentioned above to determine the effect of these foods on various diseases, such as heart disease, Type 2 diabetes, colorectal cancer, and stroke. They also assessed the impact of eating an extra portion of these foods every week. In addition to this, they also assessed the harm these foods cause on the environment. They found that these foods increase water pollution, air pollution, emission of greenhouse gases and other problems. They also studied the effect of various healthy foods, such as nuts, legumes, whole-grain cereals, vegetables and fruit, and found that these foods had a low impact on the environment.

It was found that processed and unprocessed red meat, such as beef and pork, had the worst impact on the environment. Not all animal products were as bad as others. For instance, fish does not have a significant impact on the environment, and is also beneficial to human health. Sugary drinks also have minimal or low impact on the environment, but they pose significant risks on human health. Red meat has a negative impact on the environment as discussed already.

This research shows that people should consider their dietary choices. For instance, researchers wanted to use this opportunity to convince producers and manufacturers to display the information on their labels. They wanted them to state both environmental and health impacts on their labels. The team also wanted to help consumers use this information wisely to purchase the right foods. The authors of this report concluded that it was best to replace harmful foods with healthy foods, such as dairy, grains, cereals, chicken and eggs, since they have minimal or no impact on the environment. These foods could also improve your health and reduce any harm they may cause on the environment.

It is difficult to control every aspect of what you eat, but it is only when you read such information that you can choose to adopt a healthier diet. Experts have also seen that as the population increases, more tropical areas and forests are being turned into grasslands to graze cattle and farmlands for crops. What people seem to have forgotten is that we need these areas to meet the increasing demand for food. More than 56 million acres of land are used for animal agriculture, and only four million acres are used to grow crops to feed people. Since more than 70% of the produce is fed to animals, there is very little that goes to people. It would be prudent to use the acre of land used to produce 250 pounds of beef to produce 53,000 pounds of potatoes and 50,000 pounds of tomatoes. After going through the information given in the previous chapters about food labels, you now understood that most industries merely play with words to reduce their accountability. Be wise and stay informed!

As per a study conducted by Tilman et al., (2014), the only way to overcome these issues is by leaving the animal diet behind. As the global population continues to grow, the demand for crops will increase by 120 percent by the year 2050, and it would be easier to switch to the plant-based diet now, rather than later. If this happens, the land used to graze cattle and grow crops for cattle will reduce by 1.2 billion hectares, which can be used to produce food for people.

Chapter Six:

An Easy Guide to Making the Switch

The book has shed some light on why it is important to switch to a plant-based diet, and how this not only helps the planet, but also saves lives. If you are excited to switch to a plant-based diet, there is no time like the present! Are you wondering how to start this diet? Do you have any queries about the general nutrition on this diet? Are you looking for tips on how to easily switch to this diet? Don't worry, as this is something most people worry about. It is only when you try, you will find there are ample food options for you to eat. A switch to a plant-based diet is a mature, educated, and thoughtful thing to do, especially if you are dedicated to making this shift for the animals around you and yourself.

If your reasons are strong enough, you need to be willing to go through some trial and error. It may be slightly difficult for you to explain to your family and friends why you no longer eat meat, but soon this becomes your reality.

It may have been difficult a few years ago to switch to this diet, but since the vegan trend is going strong, it is easier than ever to make the switch. Many people around you have already paved the way, all you need to do is follow their instructions to navigate through the diet.

How to Start the Diet

This section has 12 tips you can use to ease yourself into the plant-based diet. Each step will simplify your transition in a different way.

Ask Yourself "Why?"

If you have reached this chapter, you are probably right on the precipice of making some profound changes to your eating habits and lifestyle. Before you jump, take a second and focus on your goals. Ask yourself what you want to achieve when you follow this diet. Why is it important for you to switch to the diet? You may want to increase your energy, reduce the risk of developing some types of diseases, or maybe you want to save animal lives or the planet. Regardless of which reason you have, identifying it will help you move forward. If the idea of the diet excites you, it is easier to switch to this diet. Keep the reason close to your heart, so you stay motivated. Continue to read about plant-based foods regularly, so you are always learning something new about the diet. There are numerous reasons why you should avoid eating animals and animal products, and you may resonate with more and more of them over time. Watch documentaries and other videos about this diet, so you stay focused even when it becomes hard to follow the diet.

It becomes easier to follow the plant-based diet when you change the way you feel or think about meat. After going through all the chilling statistics and facts in the previous chapters, your attitude towards plant-based foods must have already changed. Try to make a connection between the animal and the meat that came from the product in the market. This makes it easier to swap between meat with other ingredients.

Some of the best documentaries to watch are:

- *Dominion*
- *Cowspiracy*
- *The Game Changers*
- *What the Health*
- *Fork Over Knives*
- *The Cove*
- *Okja*

Eat Enough

Most people are confused about how much they should eat, but the quantity differs from one person to another. The size of your meals when you follow a plant-based diet depends on what you used to eat before you made the switch. If you used to follow a protein-rich diet, high in processed foods and animal products, you need to increase your intake when you switch to a plant-based diet.

Legumes, vegetables, fruits, and grains have fewer calories when compared to meat, cheese, butter, and eggs. This is especially true when you focus on lower fat plant-based foods and whole foods. So, you can load up on fresh fruit, salads, beans, quinoa, and baked potatoes. If you cannot eat large portions, replace some of the fruit and raw vegetables with seeds, pasta, avocado, or tofu, so you get enough nutrients and calories. Of course, if you are trying to lose weight, it's a win-win for you as you will naturally eat fewer calories on a plant-based diet.

If you have trouble with controlling your hunger, switching to a whole food plant-based diet will make it easier for you. Since the diet has a high water and fiber content, it becomes easier to feel full, and maintain a healthy weight. You must eat to your heart's content, especially if you come from a restrictive eating background. Never deprive yourself. If you stick to this diet, your body will get used to the change in food volumes.

It is important to remember that everybody has a different caloric intake, and it is best to track your intake when you begin the diet. This helps you understand the different types of food you can and cannot eat. Try to restrict your caloric intake to around(add) 1,600 calories each day, and focus only on your natural hunger.

Buy Healthy Foods

The idea is simple: You can't eat something if you don't have it around you or haven't bought it. So, create an environment in your house and ensure that all the food you buy follows your goals. Before you switch to the diet, go through your pantry and get rid of food you no longer want to eat. You can either toss the food out or give it to someone who still includes it in their diet. Do not keep any food in your pantry simply because you bought it or because you think it may go to waste. Once you clean the pantry, go to the grocery store and buy potatoes, rice, nuts, beans, fruits, and vegetables, so you can always prepare healthy snacks and meals. Your main source of will be starches, such as pumpkin, legumes, whole grains, and potatoes, so make sure you have enough of these at home. You can either buy fresh or frozen produce, depending on your preference. These foods are unprocessed and healthy, and have a long shelf life. Make a conscious choice to purchase only healthy and wholesome ingredients. Once you have all the required ingredients, you can experiment with all the delicious recipes coming up in this book.

Keep Snacks Ready

When you follow the plant-based diet, you certainly won't be going hungry since. The nutritious and filling options are endless. But, what can you do if you get hungry when you are out? It is best to carry healthy snacks with you at all times, so you avoid the temptation to grab a convenient animal-based highly processed food. You can always carry a box of nuts, vegan bars, energy balls, or fresh fruit. If you have time every morning, you can make a grain-based salad, wraps, or sandwiches. Alternatively, you can also carry a box of leftover food.

Some other tips would be to grab a bite to eat before you leave the house, or pick up some plant-based snacks when you are on your way.

Swap Food Slowly

You may be eager to switch to this diet, but do not dive right into it. It is better to take a gentle approach. Even if it sounds like a simple change, your body isn't used to this new eating pattern. Therefore, give yourself some time to get used to the diet. So, instead of restricting what you eat, you should replace it. Add more plant-based food to your diet. If you used to eat animal-based or processed food, swap some of those for healthy alternatives. For example, use tofu instead of cottage cheese and chicken, avocado instead of butter and lentils, and mixed beans instead of lamb or beef. Use whole grain spaghetti instead of white flour spaghetti, have fruit as snacks and use dates instead of white sugar. You can always increase your intake of plant-based foods by replacing the stuff you no longer want to eat.

This section provides super simple swaps, so get your grocery list and pen ready!

Avocado mash instead of butter

Butter has cholesterol and pure saturated fat, which means it does not have any micronutrients. This ingredient adds 102 calories to your intake per tbsp. Butter, like many other animal products, increases the risk of developing cardiovascular diseases. You may also gain unwanted pounds. If you use the same quantity of mashed, sliced, or ripe avocado on your bread, you may only increase your caloric intake by 22 calories. This means you do not consume any saturated fats, and also eat small amounts of vitamins, minerals, and fiber. Avocado is referred to as nature's butter, and for the right reasons. Avocado toast will be your preferred go-to in no time.

Whole Fruit Instead of Smoothies or Juice

Juices and smoothies have gained a great reputation and popularity over the last few years. Most people choose to drink juices and smoothies instead of eating any fruit. If you want to lose weight, you should consider eating whole fruits, so you can better satiate your cravings and hunger. When you blend fruit, you destroy fiber, and your blood sugar reacts very differently to juices when compared to chewing and eating fruit. Your body does not detect liquid calories, which makes it hard to curb your hunger, especially since there is no fiber in the juice. It is easy to make a smoothie with a cup of berries and three bananas. Could you imagine eating so much whole fruit as a snack? Store-bought smoothies and juices may also contain added sugar, and since these smoothies are not fresh, the micronutrients are often long gone.

Baked Potatoes Instead of Fries

This is a great example to help you understand how carbs do not increase weight. Most people avoid potatoes like the plague because of their carbohydrate and starch content, and some people cut them completely out of their diet. The truth is that potatoes are probably the only food that satiate your hunger, and don't add excessive calories. One pound of potatoes only has 340 calories, but your intake doubles when you eat a bowl of whole-grain pasta.

When you eat one pound of chicken, your caloric intake increases in calories but still doesn't have a high satiety index, unlike potatoes. This does not mean you can eat a huge portion of potatoes, since the caloric intake depends on how you prepare them. If you want to reap the benefits of potatoes, avoid using cream, cheese, butter, or oil when you cook them. One pound of fries adds 1,350 calories to your plate, but a plate of baked potatoes only add 380 calories. This is quite a difference, isn't it? You can cut potatoes into strips and season them with pepper, salt, paprika and other herbs and spices. Bake them in the oven without adding any oils or cheese.

Oats Instead of Breakfast Cereal and Granola

Another meal that is often hyped is granola, but have you ever looked at the ingredients on the box? Granola is crunchy and delicious, but there is a lot of added sugar and oil. Since some granola also has added fruit and nuts, the dish has a higher number of calories. These sugary breakfasts are refined and processed and do not keep your hunger at bay. You can always make granola at home without any added sugar, oil, or other unhealthy ingredients. You can use small portions of dried nuts and seeds to sweeten it. Alternatively, you can eat a bowl of rolled oats. Oatmeal does not have too many calories, and you can always control what you add to the bowl of oatmeal. This makes it one of the best breakfast choices you can make.

Almond Milk Instead of Cow Milk

These food swaps may not be new to you, but there are numerous reasons why you should choose almond milk instead of cow milk, which this book has touched upon. Even if you drink one cup of fat-free cow milk, your caloric intake increases by 83 calories. A cup of unsweetened almond milk only has 36 calories, and this is not only a great substitute but adds an interesting flavor. You can also make almond milk at home, and hence this is a cheaper alternative. According to studies and surveys conducted by the NIH, close to 65% of the world's population can no longer digest lactose after infancy. This means there is a chance that dairy products cause various troubles. You can overcome various digestive and skin issues if you abstain from dairy products for a few days or weeks. I'd say it's worth a try! If you want to buy almond milk in the supermarket, check to make sure it isn't fortified.

Potato Crust Instead of Flour

Whole grains are delicious, healthy, and filling, which is why these ingredients are best for weight loss. If you roast and grind these grains and legumes into flour, the calorie density will go up. That said, you can always make many of your favorite meals without using any flour. You may still want to eat pizza, and now you can without using flour.

You can satiate your starch craving by using a mix of mashed potato and cauliflower, for the crust. You can then top the pizza with beans and any kind of vegetables. Do not use fatty and caloric-dense animal products on the pizza crust if you don't want to ruin the effort of making this healthy crust. Do not use cheese, but try nutritional yeast instead.

Cinnamon and Fruit Instead of Sugar

It is important to avoid eating too much sugar both for your waistline and your overall health. Refined sugars are all the same, regardless of whether you use brown sugar, white sugar, coconut sugar, honey, or agave syrup. These sugars act the same in your body, and do not offer any nutrition. Processed food has a lot of refined and added sugar, and therefore, you should avoid these foods if you want to lose weight. You can sweeten home-cooked meals using fruit instead of sugar. Mangoes, bananas, and dates get the job done especially well. These are the sweetest fruits, and keep in mind that dried fruit is always sweeter and denser. Cinnamon makes food sweeter, too and makes a snappy addition to your morning oatmeal. You can increase the sweetness of apples, bananas, or plums by baking or cooking them.

Roasted Edamame or Chickpeas Instead of Nuts

Nuts are generally considered good for your health. Nuts are always better for you instead of meat, eggs, and cheese because they have more fiber and less saturated fat—not to mention the added benefits that choosing plants over animal products has for the environment. That said, if you want to lose weight faster and more easily, limit how often you snack on them. You can add some nuts and fruit to your salad and oatmeal bowls, but don't inhale a whole pack in one sitting. Instead of eating roasted and salted nuts, you can roast edamame and chickpeas with spices and no oil instead. Alternatively, you can bake them. One cup of roasted edamame and chickpeas has 200 calories, but a cup of mixed nuts has more than four times this number.

Applesauce Instead of Butter or Oil

You can use avocado instead of butter when you eat toast, but what do you do when you need to bake cake? Avocado is never a perfect substitute for butter, but luckily there is a baking alternative to butter and oil. You can use applesauce instead of butter when you bake your next muffins! This ingredient is not only low in calories but it also adds a fruity flavor to the dish.

Cauliflower Sauce Instead of Cheese Sauce

This may sound a bit strange to you, but I promise this is the best alternative to a cheese sauce. Even if you do not like this vegetable on its own, you can still use it as the perfect base for creamy sauce. You only need to add some simple ingredients and the right spices to have a low-calorie, homemade and plant-based sauce. You can use this sauce for vegetables or pasta. Most creamy sauces are rich and fatty, and these add calories to your pasta dish. A plant-based sauce made from cooked potatoes, carrots, or cauliflower lowers the caloric density of the entire dish. You can also use nutritional yeast, as it increases the creamy texture of the dish.

Low-Fat and Oil-Free Salad Dressings

Most people eat salads when they want to lose weight, but this isn't a fool-proof method. Yes, leafy grains are very nutritious and are also low in calories, but only when you haven't added too much olive oil. Olive oil is loaded with fat. And though the fats aren't saturated, one tbsp of olive oil still packs 120 calories. This is likely more than all the greens you include in the salad. Opt for oil-free and low-fat salad dressing if you can. You can also try vinegar, fruit, beans, mustard, seeds, or avocado to spice up your greens. You can also try to make your own pesto at home, which can be both low in fat and still creamy. This may become your new favorite food!

Mustard or Hummus Instead of Mayo

Most people avoid bread because of its carbohydrates. According to many, bread makes it hard to lose weight. But how bad do you think a slice of bread with mayonnaise is for you? It is true that white flour has more calories when compared to grains, but the number of calories are lower in bread when compared to mayonnaise. Mayonnaise has the same number of calories as butter. Just one ounce of mayonnaise has 200 calories! It is very easy to eat mayonnaise because it adds a quick punch of flavor to sandwiches. If you swap mayonnaise with mustard or hummus on your bread, you only consume 50 calories.

Beans Instead of Meat

This is probably the tastiest swap, especially if you love chili. If you already follow a plant-based diet, you can use this method to get your family to transition along with you. Beans are a great way to aid in weight loss since they are low in fat and extremely versatile. These ingredients are filled with slow-releasing complex carbs, and are a great source of protein. Beans have less than 50% of the calories than meat and are still super filling.

Sweet Potato Toast Instead of Bread

We did talk about the difference between flour products, such as pizza bases and bread, and potatoes. This is another twist you can consider trying. Cut sweet potatoes into cubes or slices and place them in the toaster oven. Leave them to cook in the oven until they turn soft. You can enjoy these slices instead of bread. A whole, medium sweet potato is equivalent to one slice of bread, considering the calorie count. Just like with your sliced bread, you can add delicious toppings. Try mashed chickpeas, avocado, and fruit on top of the sweet potato for a delicious and nutritious snack or lunch!

Eat a Plant-Based Breakfast

It can be daunting to jump to three vegan meals every day, especially if you are just starting out. So, it is best to start off with one at a time. I suggest beginning with breakfast as it is super easy to veganize. Nothing says tasty and healthy like a bowl of oatmeal loaded with fruit! It is an easy, nutritious, and delicious way to begin your day. If oatmeal isn't your jam, don't worry; you've got many more vegan breakfast options. Consider chia pudding, pancakes, avocado and potato toast, tofu scramble, or peanut butter and jelly sandwiches for your morning meal. There are even more vegan breakfast options to choose from, and we will look at some of these recipes later in the book. Plant-based breakfast inspires you to continue on your healthy path throughout the day, making switching to healthy vegan lunch more attainable. When you are confident that you can stick to a plant-based breakfast regularly, move on to tackling your lunch, and finally dinner. You should continue to do this until all your snacks and meals are transformed into plant-based alternatives. If the idea of food preparation is making you nervous, the easiest thing to do is make extra for lunch, so you have something to eat for dinner.

Educate Yourself

There are a lot of myths and misinformation about the plant-based diet, and some of these have been covered in the book. Unfortunately, there are more out there and many people hastily criticize this diet choice. The modern diet focuses on the consumption of animal products since they are rich in protein and healthy fat. Therefore, it is understandable that people around you may not like the idea of a plant-based diet. So, before you try to change their minds about the diet, get your facts right. The Academy of Nutrition and Dietetics, and other such organizations, have stated that a vegan diet is healthy for all stages of life if planned correctly. Many dieticians and doctors recommend this diet to reduce the symptoms of chronic diseases.

Apart from the articles and documentaries mentioned above, you can grab books about plant-based eating and veganism, like this book. Alternatively, you can go through some blogs written by people following this diet so you are prepared to educate others who question your choices.

Find a Support Group

Human beings like to socialize; this is especially true when adjusting to a new lifestyle. It is extremely useful to surround yourself with people who have the same beliefs and health goals as you. If you switch to the diet alone, it becomes hard to organize, justify, and remind yourself why you should make the effort day after day. You may even convince yourself that the diet is not worth it anymore. If you do not have support at home, from your friends, coworkers, or family, it is recommended that you reach out to someone online. Search for virtual forums, so you stay motivated to continue this diet. One of the best places to start doing this is Facebook, since there are numerous plant-based and vegan groups, and some of these groups may even be in your area.

It is invaluable if you have someone to talk to about this diet, especially if you need to find a specific product, rant, or ask for help. You can use other platforms like Meetup if you want to get in touch with like-minded people in person. When people around you see your progress, they may also want to switch to the plant-based diet. So, let your results speak for themselves, and connect with people who feel the same way.

Have the Right Equipment

You need to have the right kitchen tools at home, such as a cutting board, baking sheets, nonstick pan, sharp knives, and pots. You should also have a personal or immersion blender, spiralizer, and pressure cooker. The collection of these appliances lets you create a variety of meals to keep you inspired and satisfied on your plant-based journey.

You don't have to break the bank by buying all of these machines brand new. Ask friends and family if they have any spare equipment they can lend you. Check out Marketplace and second-hand sources, too. If you become a frequent user, then you can invest in the new equipment later on. Some online stores, like Amazon, have amazing deals, so keep an eye out or set up an alert for your desired appliance.

Create New Habits Gently

When you are kind to yourself, you learn to not beat yourself up if you feel you aren't doing things the right way or haven't met your goals yet. Make sure to keep your visions and dreams close by and always work towards them. But be gentle with yourself. Allow yourself to accept your current position and take the process step-by-step, acknowledging the reality of the journey. You must remember that your thoughts have a significant impact both on your reality and perception. It all comes down to developing new eating habits. This is the only way the diet begins to feel like second nature to you.

When you put yourself under pressure and put yourself down, it can cause a spiral of negative events and beliefs. You should not adjust your expectations or forget about the bigger picture, but do this according to your expectations. You can succeed only when you become your biggest supporter and fan. So, go back to some of the points mentioned above, and take care of every meal before you switch to this diet.

It is best to put a vegan or vegetarian cookbook together, so it becomes easier to discover and experience the diversity these meals offer. You must understand that being a vegan is not only about eating rice and salads, but there is a ton of flavor and color you can include to your meals. The possibilities are nearly endless!

Keep Things Exciting and Fun

When you dabble in a plant-based diet, you should always push your boundaries and comfort zone a bit. There are many dishes you have never heard of or tried. Next time you go to the supermarket, look at the assortment of vegetables, fruit, lentils, beans, nuts, seeds, and grains. Instead of mindlessly reaching for "the regulars" choose a few ingredients that you have never eaten before or that look interesting to you. You can also seek out unique meals and ideas on the Internet, for your next lunch adventure. You can even use snacks to expand your horizons. There are new plant-based packaged snack options being released daily!

Commit to the Diet

You now have a solid foundation for your new lifestyle, and therefore, it is time to commit to the diet. You can take a few days, weeks, or months to put everything into action. Regardless of how long it takes you to get into it, you must ensure you follow through with the plan you develop. You should clear out your pantry and kitchen, have all the staples on hand, and strive to enjoy every bite of every meal. Maintain a list of favorite plant-based snacks and recipes, so you can easily refer to them to support your diet. You can also follow some vegan plans and groups on social media if you need additional inspiration along the way. This will help you feel a little less alone. It is only when you commit yourself in these ways that you can transform easily and completely. Put in the time and effort and you will recognize the benefits of the diet.

You may want to jump into the plant-based diet overnight, and this may work for a few people, but it will take a lot of willpower and improvisation if you want to stay on track. This change is overwhelming, and some may fall off the wagon. You might temporarily go back to eating junk food, processed food, and animal products. Your likelihood to go off track is dependent on which type of diet you are coming from. For instance, it is easier to transition if you are already following a diet rich in legumes, grains, fruits, and vegetables. It will be more of a challenge if you are coming from a diet rich in meat and processed foods. Either way, it is crucial to gently ease into the diet, so you do not add too much pressure and lose all motivation entirely.

Choosing the Right Diet

As you may know, there are variations of plant-based diets. This might make it difficult for a person to know exactly which one to go for. Some people choose to exclude all animal products while others may decide to eat some of them sparingly. Others may only restrict specific types of animal meat. This section looks at four different types of plant-based diets and also discusses some variations of these diets to help you adopt the right diet for you.

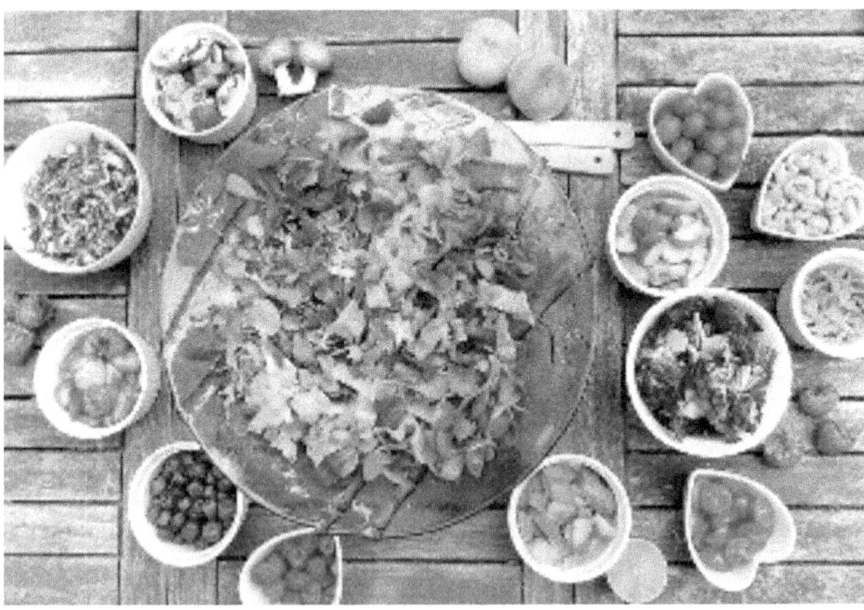

Vegan Diet

A vegan diet is a plant-based diet wherein you must avoid the consumption of animal products and byproducts, including eggs, dairy, fish, and meat. You may decide to follow this diet for numerous reasons, including environmental issues, health benefits, and animal welfare concerns. A vegan diet is a common plant-based diet, and many vegans also abstain from the use of animal products, such as wool and leather. Some examples of the food allowed on this diet include:

- All types of fruit
- Legumes
- All types of grains
- All starchy and non-starchy vegetable options
- Nuts and seeds
- Olive oil, vegetable oil, coconut oil, walnut oil, avocado oil
- Spices
- Herbs

Some types of foods you cannot eat on a vegan diet are:

- Meat, such as seafood, lamb, fish, poultry, pork, beef, meat-based sauces and broths
- Dairy products, such as yogurt, cheese, cream, milk, ice cream, casein, lactose and whey
- Eggs

- Fish oil, mayonnaise, butter, tallow, and lard
- Other products, such as fish sauce, honey, gelatin, Vitamin D3 supplements, food coloring, additives, and bee pollen

Though this diet is included in the list of plant-based diets, there is still a debate on whether it should be included. Since the definition of a plant-based diet is vague, there is no way to describe the diet using one word. People follow different dietary patterns even in this category. There are some people who follow a plant-based, whole foods diet. This diet emphasizes on the consumption of minimally processed or whole plant foods, and excludes the consumption of sugars, vegetable oils and refined grains. Since a vegan diet is restrictive, it is difficult for some people to obtain the required nutrition, and thus may need to include fortified foods and supplements.

Vegetarian Diet

This is one of the most popular forms of a plant-based diet, and it is less restrictive when compared to a vegan diet. These diets allow the consumption of all the foods allowed on a vegan diet, and also exclude seafood, meat, and fish. A vegetarian diet, however, may allow the consumption of dairy products and eggs depending on the type of vegetarian diet you wish to follow.

Since a vegetarian diet is flexible, it always includes various types of foods, and there may be no need to consume fortified foods or take nutritional supplements to meet your nutritional needs. This, however, is dependent on the individual, and in most cases your need for supplements depends on the choices you make. There are three types of vegetarian diets.

Lacto-Ovo Vegetarian

A lacto-ovo diet is one where you should avoid eating meat. You are still allowed to eat eggs and dairy products, however. This type of diet is often referred to as a vegetarian diet. One of the many reasons why people prefer a lacto-ovo diet is to improve their health, but they may also choose to follow this diet as a matter of preference or due to humanitarian and environmental concerns.

Ovo Vegetarian

An ovo vegetarian diet includes eggs, but it prohibits the consumption of dairy products, including cream, yogurt, butter, ice cream, cheese, and milk. People may choose to follow this diet if they have any intolerances or allergies to dairy. They may also choose to follow this diet if they do not like dairy products or are aware of the environmental reasons for avoiding dairy products.

Lacto Vegetarian

This is another variation of a vegetarian diet, but you can eat dairy products. You, however, cannot eat any food that includes eggs, such as mayonnaise, egg whites, whole eggs, or any baked goods that use eggs. There are numerous reasons why people may decide to follow this specific type of diet, including an aversion to eggs, animal welfare, or environmental concerns.

Pescatarian Diet

This diet is another plant-based diet, and is referred to by some as a vegetarian diet, despite allowing animal products. You are only allowed to consume seafood, fish and shellfish, but no other meat. The pescatarian diet, like other vegetarian diets, is based on plant-based foods, and some pescatarians also eat eggs and dairy products, but there are others who do not.

People who eat fish, eggs, and dairy follow the lacto-ovo pescatarian diet, but there is no clear segregation between these subtypes. Most people follow this diet if they want to increase their intake of omega-3 fatty acids and quality protein. Others choose to follow this diet for humanitarian reasons, environmental sustainability, and animal welfare. If you choose to follow this diet, you must be mindful about your intake of seafood and fish. It is important to remember that seafood may also be contaminated with numerous heavy metals that can lead to blood toxicity.

Predatory or large fish are higher in the food chain, and thus may accumulate numerous toxins, such as mercury and lead, which can have a negative impact on your health, especially if you increase your intake. Therefore, it is best to consume a variety of different types of fish and limit your intake of seafood and high-mercury fish, such as swordfish, escolar, tuna, shark, and marlin.

Arctic char, sardines, herring, salmon, rainbow trout, and mackerel have lower quantities of mercury, and are thus safer options. If you want to minimize this risk further, choose fish that have been caught or raised sustainably. Pregnant women and children should avoid fish and seafood to reduce the negative effects of mercury on their health. At the very least, pregnant women should consider limiting their consumption to 12 ounces per week. A balanced and well-planned pescatarian diet ensures that you meet your daily nutritional needs, thereby reducing your body's dependency on fortified foods and supplements. This diet, like every other diet, is unique to individuals and the choices they make when they follow this diet.

Semi-Vegetarian or Flexitarian Diet

This diet is the most flexible form of a plant-based diet, and it does not prohibit the consumption of animal-based products. The foundation of this diet is based on small proportions of fish, meat, eggs, plants, and dairy, but the main focus should always be on choosing plant-based products when possible. You can include animal-based products depending on your caloric and nutritional requirements. It was predicted that this type of diet will be the largest diet trend in the year 2020, and this does not come as a surprise. A semi-vegetarian or flexitarian diet is appealing to those who want to move from a meat or animal-product based diet to a plant-based diet, but are unable to take the leap into following a vegan or vegetarian diet abruptly.

This diet does not have the same rules as other plant-based diets, but has the same benefits. Some people use this diet to make it easier for them to follow a plant-based diet, such as a vegetarian or vegan diet. That said, there are some who use this diet to maximize their caloric and nutritional intake from plants, while they enjoy eating the foods they like. Most people across the globe already follow this diet, and they don't even know it.

Chapter Seven:

Mistakes to Avoid

We can't ignore the numerous benefits of a balanced vegan or vegetarian diet, including:

- Better control over blood sugar levels
- Weight loss
- Decreased risk and symptoms of heart diseases
- Lower risk of cancer

We have covered the abundance of benefits in detail already. That said, it can become difficult to maintain a balanced vegetarian diet when striving to meet your individual nutrient requirements. This chapter covers some mistakes people make when they follow this diet, and also leaves you with some tips to avoid making the same errors.

Assuming Vegetarian and Vegan Products Are Healthier

Some people don't realize that food products are not necessarily, by default, healthier simply because the product is labeled vegan or vegetarian. For instance, most people switch to almond milk and avoid drinking cow milk. Almond milk is enriched with several minerals and vitamins and is low in calories. 0.8 grams per kilogram of bodyweight is the ideal intake of protein. Almond milk is a healthier alternative to dairy, but be mindful of the almond milk you consume. Most of the processed variants available in the market are filled with sugar, additives, and preservatives. None of these ingredients are healthy. Whenever you opt for any vegan products, carefully read the labels and nutritional facts.

Some vegetarian products, such as meat alternatives, vegetable burgers, and nuggets are processed, and include numerous artificial ingredients. So, they are not inherently healthier when considering this.

These processed alternatives may be vegetarian or vegan, but they might also be high in calories. They potentially lack nutrients, protein, and fiber, too. While these products may make it easier for you to transition into a vegetarian or vegan diet, it is best to take note of the nutrition labels, and only consume them in small quantities while increasing your intake of whole foods.

Not Consuming Enough Vitamin B12

Vitamin B12 is an extremely important nutrient, and it has several roles to play. It helps in the creation of DNA and red blood cells, among many other processes. It is unfortunate that the main sources of this vitamin are various animal products, such as milk products, shellfish, meat, eggs, and poultry. It is for this reason most people following this diet are at a risk of developing a Vitamin B12 deficiency, which can cause memory problems, numbness, and fatigue. This deficiency can also cause megaloblastic anemia, which is a condition where you have very few red blood cells. Most people do not identify the symptoms of Vitamin B12 until the damage becomes irreversible. Don't give up, however. There are many foods and supplements you can take to meet your B12 requirements. For starters, some forms of edible algae and fortified foods are good sources of Vitamin B12. The next chapter has a list of supplements you can use to increase your B12 intake.

Eating Cheese Instead of Meat

If you are not on a vegan diet, many people will replace meat with cheese. This swap works very well for pastas, sandwiches, salads, and various casseroles. Cheese does have a lot of vitamins, minerals, and substantial protein. However, cheese cannot replace a lot of other nutrients found in meat. For example, an ounce of beef has at least twice the amount of zinc and four times the amount of iron when compared to one ounce of cheese. Cheese, however, has fewer calories when compared to meat, but also has a lower protein content. Chicken contains at least 80% more protein than cheese, but has 2.5 times the calories contained in cheese. You cannot simply replace meat with cheese and call it a day. Instead, include a variety of plant foods to your diet, so you meet your nutritional needs in a more well-rounded way. Tempeh, quinoa, beans, nuts, lentils, and chickpeas are excellent additions.

Reducing Your Caloric Intake

As you know, when you follow a vegetarian or vegan diet, you must avoid certain foods and food groups, and therefore, it can be challenging for you to meet your daily caloric needs. Vegetarians and vegans often eat fewer calories when compared to people who eat plants and meat. According to a study by Clarys et al., vegetarians had a higher caloric intake when compared to vegans, but they still consumed fewer calories when compared to people who ate plants and meat. The study measured the nutritional intake of 1,500 people, including people who ate meat once a week, those who ate plants and meat, vegetarians who ate fish, vegans, and vegetarians. This study found that vegans ate very few calories (Clarys et al., 2014). Your caloric intake is your body's source of energy, and your body has a daily requirement without which it cannot function. When you restrict your caloric intake too much, it can lead to numerous side effects, including slower metabolism, nutrient deficiencies, and fatigue.

Reducing Your Water Intake

Regardless of which diet you follow, you must ensure you drink a lot of water, and this is especially true for those whose fiber intake is higher. If you follow a vegetarian diet, your fiber intake may be higher since you are loading up on vegetables, legumes, and whole grains in your diet. People who ate both plants and meat ate at least 27 grams of fiber regularly, while vegetarians and vegans ate 34 grams and 41 grams, respectively. It is for this reason you must drink more water, so you can make it easier for your body to digest fiber to prevent various digestive issues, such as constipation, gas, and bloating. It is also critical for you to increase your fiber intake, as fiber reduces the risk of stroke, obesity, heart disease, and diabetes. According to the guidelines issued by the American Heart Association, people should eat at least 25 grams of fiber every day. You must drink water when you are thirsty, and ensure you drink enough to stay hydrated throughout the day as your fiber increases.

Not Eating Enough Iron

Meat has a large share of vitamins and minerals, especially iron. For instance, one serving of ground beef increases your intake of iron by 14%. Meat is rich in heme iron, which your body can absorb easily. Plant foods are rich in non-heme iron, and your body has difficulty in absorbing this iron easily. This form of iron is present in various fruit, cereals, beans, and vegetables. It is for this reason most vegetarians are at the risk of developing iron deficiencies, such as anemia. This condition is where your body cannot produce red blood cells, and some symptoms include dizziness, fatigue, and shortness of breath.

Having said that, if you follow a well-planned vegetarian diet, you can include iron-rich plant food, so you easily meet your daily iron needs. If you are a vegan or vegetarian, you must ensure you increase your intake of iron rich food, including fortified cereals, seeds, beans, lentils, leafy greens, and oats. It is also good to pair iron rich food with foods rich in calcium and Vitamin C to enhance your body's ability to absorb non-heme iron. Vitamin C is found in many vegetables and fruits, so it is best to include a salad, piece of fruit, and side dish to increase iron absorption.

Avoiding Whole Foods

Food is not automatically better because it is vegan or vegetarian, as we've touched on earlier. There are many processed foods in the supermarket that are free of animal and meat products, but they still don't add any nutritional value to your diet. Instead of eating processed food, increase your consumption of whole foods, such as whole grains, fruits, and vegetables. These foods give you the valuable vitamins, antioxidants, and minerals and also help to prevent nutrient deficiencies and improve metabolism. A study conducted by (Barr et al., 2010) found that whole-food and processed-food meals have an implication on your daily energy expenditure, as people burn more calories when they eat whole foods. The team monitored the metabolism of the participants before and after they ate the meals, with either whole or processed food. Both these groups felt full after the meal, but the group that ate whole foods burned more calories than the group that ate processed food. If you want to include more whole foods in your diet, you should swap refined grains for whole grains, and restrict your intake of processed food. You can also try to add more fruit and vegetables to your snacks and meals throughout the day.

Not Eating Enough Calcium

Your body needs enough calcium to keep your teeth and bones strong. Calcium also improves the functions of the immune and nervous system and helps your muscles work better. Since calcium helps to strengthen your bones, a deficiency can lead to osteoporosis. If you develop this condition, it can make your bones porous and weak. It may also increase the number of bone fractures. Calcium is found in numerous plant foods, and dairy products aren't the only source of calcium. As mentioned in the previous chapters, dairy products aren't as healthy as the dairy industry's intensive marketing campaigns would have us believe. From increasing the risk of certain types of diseases to the traces of harmful pesticides and antibiotics, dairy products aren't beneficial to your health. Also, there isn't any scientific research to back the claims about milk helping bone health. You must monitor your calcium intake which means you must increase your intake of high-calcium plant-based foods.

Some plant foods rich in calcium are collard greens, bok choy, broccoli, kale, oranges, almonds, and figs. You can also increase your intake of fortified foods if you are aiming to increase your calcium intake. Include a few servings of these ingredients to your snacks and meals, so you fulfill your calcium requirement in the healthiest way possible.

Not Planning Your Meals

Regardless of whether you dine out or cook at home, you must plan your meals in advance if you follow a vegan or vegetarian diet. It is especially useful to create a meal plan, when easing the transition from a meat-based diet to a plant-based diet. A meal plan makes it easier to switch to this diet, and also helps you ensure your diet remains nutritious and balanced. If you travel often or eat out frequently, you can still plan your meals in advance. Some restaurants have very few vegetarian or vegan choices. Take time to preview the menu ahead of time, so you don't make a hasty and unhealthy decision on the spot. Meal plans are incredibly useful, but don't simply copy and paste your plan from week to week until the end of time. Keep your eyes open for exciting, new vegetarian recipes every week and make tweaks every now and again.

Not Meeting Protein Requirements

Protein is an important macronutrient to include in your diet, since your body uses it to create enzymes, produce hormones, and build and repair tissue. Protein reduces cravings, satisfies hunger, and increases muscle mass. Nutritionists and dieticians recommend that adults should eat at around 0.36 g of protein for every pound of your weight. So if you are 140 lb, you should aim for around 50 g of protein. That said, always follow personalized recommendations from a doctor.

When you follow a vegetarian diet, you should be conscious about the food you eat, and increase your consumption of high-protein food. This is the only way to meet your protein requirement. There are numerous plant foods you can consume to fulfill this protein requirement. For instance, a cup of cooked chickpeas or lentils has at least 20 grams of protein. If you increase your intake of tempeh, tofu, nut butters, beans, lentils and whole nuts, you can easily meet your protein requirements. Make sure to include at least two or more of these foods in every meal, to make meeting your requirements balanced throughout the day.

Not Eating Enough Fatty Acids

Omega-3 fatty acids are important for the body because they alleviate inflammation, reduce the symptoms of dementia and control blood sugar and triglycerides. These acids have Eicosapentaenoic acid (EPA) and docosahexaenoic acid (DHA), which are extremely good for health. Plant-based foods contain ALA or alpha-linolenic acid, which is another type of fatty acid. Your body, however, has to convert ALA into EPA and DHA, so it can use it. According to a study on the synthesis of long chain fatty acids in adults done by Plourde and Cunnane (2007), your body cannot convert at least 90% of the ALA from plant food to DHA and EPA. Therefore, when you follow a vegetarian diet, you must consume ALA rich food and also eat plant-based supplements. Some plant foods rich in ALA are walnuts, chia seeds, flaxseeds, perilla oil, hemp seeds, and Brussels sprouts. You should try to include at least a few servings of these foods regularly to help you meet your omega-3 requirements.

Increasing Your Carb Intake

When people make a switch from a meat-based diet to a plant-based diet, they often replace meat with carbohydrates. It is unfortunate that most people eat crackers, bread, pasta, bagels, and cakes instead of meat, especially if their diet is poorly planned or they are just starting out. Refined grains are often stripped of their nutritional value and beneficial fiber during their processing. Fiber helps to ward off chronic diseases, and this keeps you full. Fiber also helps to reduce the absorption of sugar thereby controlling the levels of blood sugar. According to the study done on the consumption of noodles and rice and their connection with insulin resistance and Hyperglycemia in Asians (Zuñiga et al., 2014), the risk of developing diabetes increases due to a higher intake of refined carbs, which also increases belly fat. If you want to maximize your nutrient intake, you should avoid the consumption of refined grains, such as pasta, white rice and white bread for whole grains, such as brown rice, oats, buckwheat, and quinoa. You must also ensure you pair these foods with whole grains, fruit, legumes and vegetables, so you maintain a nutritious and balanced diet.

A balanced vegetarian diet is both delicious and healthy. It also protects the environment. These diets have the potential to lead to some health problems and nutrient deficiencies, but only if you do not plan them well. Make sure to eat plenty of unprocessed and whole foods to ensure you consume the right nutrients. That said, some might benefit from taking various supplements, which we will cover in the next section.

Essential Supplements for a Plant-Based Diet

A plant-based diet isn't nutritionally deficient if you pay attention to the food you consume. However, there are some essential nutrients you should pay special attention to as your plant-based diet has removed all animal products and their potential nutritional benefits. To ensure that your body gets all the nutrients it needs, here are some common vegan supplements you should pay attention to.

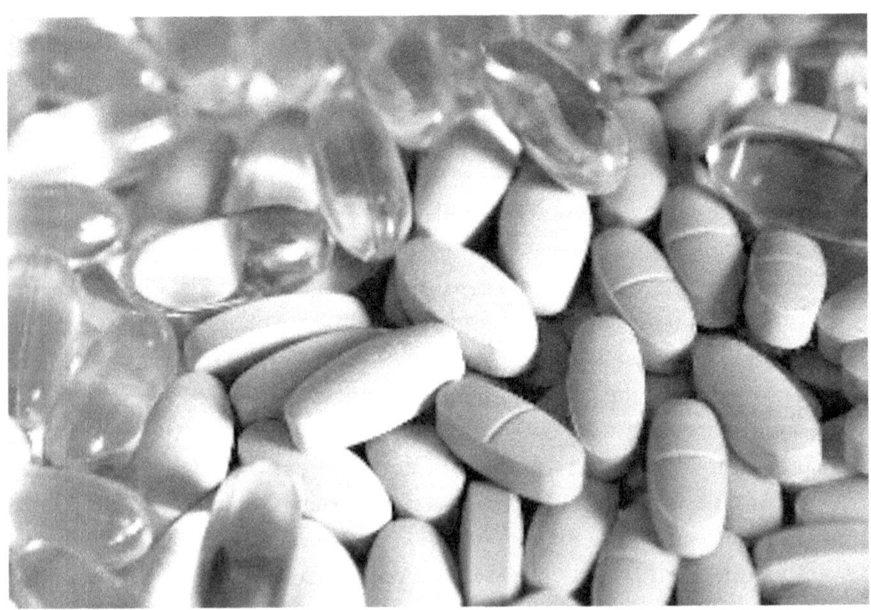

Vitamin B12

The most common supplement vegans should include in the diet is vitamin B12. It's quintessential to maintain various bodily processes. It helps metabolize proteins, produce red blood cells, and is crucial for the nervous system's health. There are limited vegan sources of this essential nutrient. Therefore, it is one of the most common vitamin deficiencies in vegans. Before you take a supplement, remember, absorption and utilization of this essential vitamin differs from one individual to another. Even meat-eaters can develop this deficiency if the body cannot optimally absorb vitamin B12. Age is another factor that must be considered because the body's ability to absorb it decreases as you age.

Therefore, it is prudent for all vegans and vegetarians to check their vitamin B12 levels regularly. Before you make any dietary changes, consult a dietician or a physician if you have any pre-existing medical conditions or health problems. The best source for vitamin B12 is through nori, as per many studies. Nori is a seaweed with high levels of vitamin B12 and other vital nutrients such as polyunsaturated fatty acids and iron. Another simple solution available is to include nutritional yeast to your daily diet. This cheesy and nutty flavored ingredient is fortified with the vitamins a vegan diet is often lacking.

Apart from nori, there are a variety of vitamin B12 fortified food products available on the market today, such as tofu, soy, breakfast cereals, nut milk, or even rice.

Iron

Another important nutrient you must pay attention to is iron. As with vitamin B12, anyone following a plant-based diet should regularly check their iron levels too. Iron is a vital nutrient required for developing and maintaining the health of red blood cells. Red blood cells perform an important function by carrying and supplying oxygen to different cells. There are two forms of iron: non-heme and heme iron. Any iron derived from animals is known as heme iron, and the ones derived from plants is non-heme iron. It's easier for the human body to absorb and utilize heme iron when compared with the non-heme variety. According to the study "Iron and Vegetarian Diets" (2013), anyone following a plant-based diet needs to include sufficient iron-rich foods. The best plant-based sources of iron include legumes, seeds, nuts, whole grains, dark leafy vegetables, dried fruits, and fortified foods and cereals.

The common symptoms of iron deficiency include shortness of breath, fatigue, pale skin, swelling or soreness of the tongue, dizziness, weakness, strange cravings, constant headaches, irregular heartbeat, and brittle nails. Iron deficiency is also known as anemia. You must pay attention to the iron you consume; your body's ability to absorb it also matters. Keep in mind that vitamins C deficiency reduces or hampers your body's ability to absorb and utilize iron optimally.

If you increase your vitamin C intake, it increases the body's absorption of the iron you consume. If you consume enough of these foods, you don't have to worry about an iron deficiency. However, before you start taking a supplement, always consult a doctor because excessive iron is dangerous, too.

Omega-3 Fatty Acids

Not all fats are created equally, and some fats are more beneficial than others. Unlike trans fats, which are extremely harmful, omega-3 fatty acids are healthy and helpful. Plant-based diets are usually rich in some types of omega-3 fatty acids and low in others. Omega-3 fatty acids help neurodevelopment, reduce the risk of cardiovascular diseases and rheumatoid arthritis, enhance memory and cognition, and lower the chances for developing Alzheimer's and dementia. It's also believed these helpful fatty acids can treat inflammatory bowel disease, cystic fibrosis, allergies, depression, and attention deficit hyperactivity disorder.

Alpha-Linolenic Acid or ALA is the most important omega-3 fatty acid. However, the human body cannot produce it and should be derived from the diet. According to the study of long chain PUFA n-3 and metabolism in women, conducted by (Burdge et al., 2017) the levels of EPA and DHA are relatively low in those who follow plant-based diets. EPA or Eicosapentaenoic acid and DHA or docosahexaenoic acid are two types of long-chain omega-3 fatty acids. These are non-essential omega-3 fatty acids because they can be produced by the body using ALA. EPA and DHA are often found in fish oils, microbiology, and fish. However, there are plenty of other sources of ALA, such as canola oil, soy products, and flaxseed. Supplements for EPA and DHA include Algeria oil supplements or concentrate.

Calcium

Calcium is an incredibly important nutrient because it helps maintain bone and teeth health, enables muscle functioning and maintenance, and is good for the heart's health, too. Those who follow a vegan diet might have a deficiency of this vital nutrient. According to studies, vegans have the lowest levels of calcium when compared with omnivores and vegetarians. The best sources of calcium include fortified foods, legumes, and all sorts of dark leafy vegetables. Your body needs vitamin D to absorb calcium. So, if you are deficient in vitamin D, calcium absorption is also harmed. If you plan well and consume sufficient foods as mentioned earlier, you don't have to worry about a calcium deficiency.

Vitamin D

From improving the immune system's function to regulating your mood and helping the absorption of other nutrients such as calcium, Vitamin D certainly plays a vital role in your overall health. When exposed to sufficient sunlight, your body can make the required vitamin D for its overall functioning. Ideally, your vitamin D dose can be attained by spending 15 to 20 minutes in the sun. It might not always be possible to spend time in the sun depending on the climate and weather conditions of your home. Also, before you step into the sun, wear sufficient sunscreen to prevent skin cancer. A plant-based diet doesn't include any dairy products, and the most common dietary sources of vitamin D are yogurt and milk. It is extra important to pay attention to your vitamin D levels. You can opt for vitamin D fortified cereals and include mushrooms in your favorite recipes. Ideally, taking a vitamin D supplement will suffice.

Zinc

Your immune system and body metabolism require zinc. However, there are hardly any plant-based sources of zinc. Plant-based compounds known as phytates also interfere with your body's absorption of zinc. Phytates are found in cereals and legumes. According to a study done on the effect of vegetarian diets on zinc (Foster et al., 2013), the overall levels of zinc in vegans and vegetarians are relatively low. Therefore, consult your healthcare provider and start taking a zinc supplement if required.

Vitamin K

Your body needs vitamin K for blood clotting and healing purposes. The two forms of vitamin K are K1 and K2. You can easily obtain the required dose of vitamin K1 from dark leafy green vegetables. The most common source of vitamin K2 is in egg yolks and dairy products. Since a plant-based diet is devoid of these things, you need to look for other sources. The best dietary sources of vitamin K2 are fermented foods such as unpasteurized kombucha, kimchi, plant-based kefir, raw sauerkraut, and natto. Your gut bacteria can successfully convert vitamin K1 into vitamin K2, too. As long as you consume plenty of dark green leafy vegetables, a vitamin K deficiency is highly unlikely. Include the above-mentioned fermented foods because they are incredible probiotics that help improve your gut microbiome's health.

A healthy gut microbiome makes it easier to synthesize vitamin K2 from K1 obtained through dietary sources.

Iodine

To maintain the health of your thyroid gland, monitor your iodine intake. Depending on the soil plants grow in, the iodine levels may differ. Seaweed is an amazing source of iodine. Another simple way to ensure your body gets the iodine it needs is using iodized salt. If you are still worried about your iodine intake, talk to your doctor, and take a supplement.

Chapter Eight:

Immunity Boosting Plant-Based Recipes

Orange Smoothie

Serves: 4 small or 2 large smoothies

Ingredients:

- 3–4 sweet potatoes (to become 2 cup loosely packed sweet potato puree)
- 2 tbsp almond butter (optional)
- 1 tbsp flaxseed meal or chia seeds
- ½ cup orange juice
- 2 medium bananas, sliced, frozen
- ½ tsp ground turmeric
- ½ tsp ground ginger or 2 tsp grated fresh ginger
- ½ tsp ground cinnamon
- 1 ½ cups almond milk, unsweetened
- Ice cubes, as required

Directions:

1. Firstly, bake the sweet potatoes in a preheated oven at 400 °F for about 30 minutes. You can also steam it.
2. Once cooked and cooled, peel the sweet potatoes and break into pieces. Transfer into a blender and blend until smooth.
3. Measure out 2 cups of it and use any left-overs in additional recipes.
4. Add all the ingredients for smoothie into a blender and blend until smooth.
5. Pour into glasses and serve.

Creamy Golden Milk Smoothie

Serves: 2–3

Ingredients:

- 2 cups sliced, frozen bananas
- 1 tsp ground turmeric
- ⅛ tsp pepper
- ⅛ tsp ground nutmeg
- 4 tbsp grated fresh ginger
- ½ tsp ground cinnamon
- A pinch ground cardamom
- A pinch ground cloves
- 1 ½ cups almond milk or light coconut milk, unsweetened
- Ice cubes, as required
- ½ cup fresh carrot juice (optional)

To serve:

- 2 tbsp hemp seeds (optional)

Directions:

1. Add all the ingredients into a blender and blend until smooth.
2. Serve garnished with hemp seeds.

Green PowerHouse Smoothie

Serves: 2

Ingredients:

- ½ cup chopped fresh spinach
- ½ cup pineapple chunks, fresh or frozen
- ½ banana, sliced
- ½ cup kale
- ½ cup mango, fresh or frozen
- 1 cup water

Directions:

1. Add all the ingredients into a blender and blend until smooth.
2. Add more water to dilute if desired.
3. Serve.

Healing Turmeric Golden Juice

Serves: 1

Ingredients:

<u>For turmeric paste:</u>

- ¼ cup turmeric powder
- ½ tsp cracked pepper
- ½ cup filtered water
- 3 tbsp coconut oil

For turmeric golden juice:

- 2–3 oranges
- 1 inch ginger, grated
- 1 medium carrot
- ½ tsp turmeric paste

Directions:

1. For turmeric paste: Add turmeric powder and water into a saucepan. Place the saucepan over low heat.
2. Keep stirring until a paste forms and it is well heated. Sprinkle some water on the mixture if it is very thick.
3. Stir in pepper and coconut oil. Turn off the heat.
4. Once it cools, transfer into an airtight container and refrigerate until use. It can last for about 15 days.
5. To make golden juice: Juice together oranges, ginger, and carrot paste in a juicer.
6. Pour into a glass. Add turmeric paste. Stir well and serve.

Beetroot and Cabbage Sauerkraut

Serves: 15–20

Ingredients:

- 6 cup thinly sliced cabbage
- 1 whole cabbage leaf

- ¼ - ½ cup sliced red onion (optional)
- 2 cups grated beets
- 2 tsp fine sea salt

Optional ingredients:

- 2 tsp caraway seeds
- 2–4 tsp grated ginger
- 2 cloves garlic, grated

Directions:

1. Add all the ingredients including optional ingredients (if using) into a bowl and massage the vegetables with your hands for a few minutes.
2. Cover and set aside at room temperature for a couple of hours. The vegetables, by now, will have released some water.
3. Transfer the vegetables into a large, clean glass jar. The liquid in the jar should cover the vegetables. If it does not, make some brine by mixing together 1 tsp sea salt in a cup of filtered water and pour it into the jar. You can make more as required.
4. Place the whole cabbage leaf directly on top. Press it into the liquid. If it floats above the water, keep some fermentation weights on top of the cabbage. You can also use a Ziploc bag filled with water. Close the lid and place the jar in a pan, in a cool and dry place for 3–5 days.
5. Keep a watch on it daily after three days. Bubbles will be visible. When the bubbles are on top of the liquid, the sauerkraut is ready to use. Remove the whole cabbage leaf and throw it away. Remove the weights as well.
6. Transition the jar into the refrigerator for about 9–10 hours.
7. Use as desired.

Fermented Pickles With Garlic and Dill

Serves: 8–12

Ingredients:

- 1 lb pickling cucumbers, rinsed
- 1 ½ tbsp fine sea salt
- ½ tsp fennel seeds
- ½ tsp coriander seeds
- ½ tsp peppercorns
- ½ tsp allspice
- ½ tsp mustard seeds
- ½ tsp dill seeds
- 1 fresh red chili, sliced or chili flakes to taste
- 3 cups filtered water
- 4–5 cloves garlic, peeled, sliced
- 1 tbsp chopped fresh dill
- 2 bay leaves

Directions:

1. Add some ice into a large bowl. Pour enough cold water to half fill the bowl. Add cucumbers into the chilled water bowl. Leave them for 15 minutes.
2. Pour ½ cup water into a saucepan. Place the saucepan over medium heat. Add salt and stir. When the water is warm, turn off the heat and let it cool completely.
3. Take a jar (1 quart) and add the cucumber, dill, garlic, all the spices, and bay leaf.
4. Add the salt water into the jar along with remaining water. If the cucumbers are floating, place something heavy on it like fermentation weight.

5. You can also use a Ziploc bag filled with water. Close the lid lightly and place the jar in a pan, in a cool and dry place for 3–5 days.
6. Keep a watch on it daily after 3 days. Bubbles will be visible. When the bubbles are on top of the liquid, the pickle is ready to use. Remove the weights.
7. Move the jar into the refrigerator.
8. Use as desired.

Ramen with Shiitake Broth

Serves: 2

Ingredients:

For ramen broth:

- ½ large onion, chopped
- 1 tbsp olive oil
- 2 cup water
- ½ sheet Kombu seaweed
- ½ - 1 tbsp white miso paste
- Sriracha to taste or hot chili oil
- 1 clove garlic, smashed
- 2 cup vegetable stock
- Salt to taste
- ¼ cup dried shiitake mushroom
- 1 tbsp mirin
- Pepper to taste

For ramen:

- 3–4 oz ramen noodles

- Scallions, to garnish
- Sesame seeds
- 4 oz cubed, baked tofu

For vegetables: (Use any)

- Sautéed Bok Choy or mushrooms
- Shredded or roasted carrots
- Roasted sweet potato or cauliflower or winter squash
- Kimchi

Directions:

1. Place a pot over medium-high heat. Add ½ tbsp oil. When the oil is heated, add onion and cook until translucent.
2. Lower the heat to medium. Stir in the garlic and cook until the onion turns golden brown.
3. Stir in the water, shiitake, stock mirin, and Kombu and bring to a boil.
4. Lower the heat and cook for about 20 minutes.
5. Season with salt and pepper. Turn off the heat. Blend with an immersion blender if desired. Cover and keep warm.
6. Meanwhile, cook the ramen noodles following the directions on the package.
7. Divide the ramen into 2 bowls and then the broth. Add tofu and any of the chosen vegetables. Drizzle hot sauce, chili oil. Sprinkle sesame seeds on top and serve.

Orange French Toast

Serves: 4

Ingredients:

For orange French toast:

- ¾ cup plain, nondairy milk of your choice, unsweetened
- ½ cup aquafaba (cooked liquid of chickpeas)
- ⅛ tsp ground cinnamon
- 1 tsp grated orange zest
- ¼ cup almond flour
- 1 tbsp pure maple syrup
- A pinch salt (optional)
- 4 whole-grain bread slices

For berry compete:

- ½ cup blueberries or raspberries, thaw if frozen
- ½ tsp pure maple syrup
- ¼ cup applesauce

Directions:

1. Place a wire rack on a baking sheet.
2. For orange French toast: Add all the ingredients except the bread slices into a bowl and whisk well.
3. Place a nonstick pan over medium-low heat. Take a slice of bread and dip it into the mixture for 2–3 seconds. Lift it and place it in the pan. Cook until the underside is golden brown. Flip sides and cook the other side until golden brown.
4. Slide the toast onto the wire rack.
5. Repeat the previous step and cook the remaining toasts.

6. Place the baking sheet along with the rack in the oven.
7. Bake in a preheated oven at 400 °F for 10–15 minutes until crisp.
8. To make berry compote: Add all the ingredients for berry compete into a blender. Give short pulses until chunky in texture.
9. Spoon berry compete over French toasts and serve.

Polenta With Pears and Cranberries

Serves: 2

Ingredients:

- 2 cups cooked polenta, warm
- 2 tbsp brown rice syrup
- ½ cup fresh or dried cranberries
- 1 pear, peeled, cored, diced
- ½ tsp ground cinnamon

Directions:

1. Cook the polenta following the directions on the package to make 2 cups. Divide into 2 bowls.
2. Add the remaining ingredients in a small saucepan. Place the saucepan over medium flame and cook until fruits are tender.
3. Divide into the bowls of polenta and serve.

Burrito Bowl

Serves: 1

Ingredients:

- 1 cup cooked grains of your choice
- A handful chopped romaine lettuce or cooked kale
- 1 green onion, thinly sliced
- ½ avocado, peeled, pitted, sliced
- 1 cup cooked or canned beans, drained
- 1 tomato, chopped
- ½ corn kernels, cooked
- 2–4 tbsp fresh salsa
- A handful baked tortilla chips, broken

Directions:

1. Place tortilla chips in a serving bowl. Spread the cooked grains followed by beans.
2. Top with lettuce, tomatoes, corn, onion, avocado, and finally salsa.

Chickpea Avocado Salad

Serves: 2

Ingredients:

- 2 cups cooked or canned chickpeas, drained, rinsed
- 1 clove garlic, peeled, minced
- ½ jalapeño pepper, minced

- Salt to taste
- ½ small red onion, chopped
- Zest of a lime, grated
- Juice of 2 limes
- ¼ cup chopped cilantro
- ½ avocado, peeled, pitted chopped, to top

Directions:

1. Add all the ingredients into a bowl and toss well.
2. Garnish with avocado and serve.

Easy Thai Noodles

Serves: 3

Ingredients:

- 4 oz brown rice noodles or whole-grain noodles
- 1 tbsp brown rice syrup or maple syrup
- 2 cloves garlic, minced
- ½ cup mung bean sprouts
- 2 tbsp roasted, chopped peanuts
- Lime wedges to serve
- 1 ½ tbsp soy sauce
- 1 tbsp fresh lime juice
- ½ package (from a 12 oz package) frozen Asian-style vegetables
- 1 green onion, chopped
- 2 tbsp chopped fresh cilantro

Directions:

1. Follow the directions on the package to cook the noodles.

2. Place a pan over medium heat. Add soy sauce, lime juice, 2 tbsp water, brown rice syrup, and garlic and stir well.
3. When it comes to a boil, add the Asian-style vegetables and cook until they are crisp and tender.
4. Stir in the mung bean sprouts and cooked noodles and toss well. Heat thoroughly.
5. Sprinkle green onion, cilantro, and peanuts on top.
6. Serve with lime wedges.

Easiest Vegan Teriyaki Tofu

Serves: 2–3

Ingredients:

- ½ block extra-firm tofu, cut into ¼ inch pieces
- ½ tbsp brown rice syrup
- A pinch salt
- 1 tsp vegetable oil
- ½ tsp soy sauce

Directions:

1. Place a pan over medium-high heat. Add oil and let it heat.
2. Season the tofu with salt, rubbing it in lightly. Place tofu into the pan and cook until brown on either side. Lower the heat to low heat.
3. Whisk together soy sauce and rice syrup in a bowl.
4. Pour the sauce over the tofu. Turn the tofu around in the sauce.
5. Serve hot.

Beet Chips

Serves: 4

Ingredients:

- 4 medium to large beets, peeled and sliced with a mandolin slicer
- Salt to taste
- 1 tbsp oil
- Spices of your choice
- Herbs of your choice

Directions:

1. Dry the chips by patting with paper towels.
2. Sprinkle salt and herbs over the beets. Spread it on a baking dish.
3. Bake in a preheated oven at 325 °F for 10–15 minutes until crisp.
4. Remove from the oven and cool completely. Sprinkle spices on top and serve.
5. Store leftovers in an airtight container.

Thyme Sea Salt Crackers

Serves: About 20

Ingredients:

- ¼ cup white whole wheat flour
- 1 ¼ cups all-purpose flour

- ½ tsp salt
- 3 tbsp olive oil, divided
- ½ tsp sea salt or kosher salt
- ½ tsp salt
- 1 tbsp minced fresh thyme
- 6 tbsp water

Directions:

1. Add white whole wheat flour, all-purpose flour, and salt into a bowl and stir until well incorporated.
2. Add 2 tbsp oil and water and stir constantly with a fork. The mixture is well combined when it doesn't stick when pressed with a finger or fork.
3. Dust your countertop with some flour.
4. Make 2 equal portions of the dough and shape into balls.
5. Place the dough on your countertop and roll with a rolling pin until it is ⅛ inch thick.
6. Take a 1 ½ inch cookie cutter and cut out round crackers. Place it on the baking sheet.
7. Collect the scrap dough and re-shape into a ball.
8. Roll it once again and cut out crackers. Repeat this process until there is no scrap dough left.
9. Pierce the crackers using a fork. Brush the crackers with 1 tbsp oil. Use more oil if required.
10. Add sea salt and thyme into a bowl and mix well. Sprinkle this mixture over each cracker.
11. Bake in a preheated oven at 375 °F for 9–11 minutes until the underside is light brown.
12. Cool completely and transfer into an airtight container.

Raspberry Coconut Ice Cream

Serves: 8–10

Ingredients:

- 3 cup frozen raspberries
- 8 tsp maple syrup
- 2 cup full fat coconut cream
- ⅔ cup liquid from the can of coconut cream

Directions:

1. Add all the ingredients into a blender and blend until creamy.
2. Serve right away for a soft serve consistency.
3. For firm ice cream, transfer into an airtight container and freeze until firm.

Healthy Vegan Summer Glow Bowl

Serves: 2

Ingredients:

For salad:

- ¾ cup black barley or any other grain of your choice
- 2 cup water
- ½ fennel bulb, thinly shaved
- ½ orange, peeled, separated into segments, chopped
- ½ avocado, peeled, pitted, sliced
- 1 cup blueberries

- ½ bunch watercress
- 2 tbsp thinly sliced red onion
- 2 tbsp chopped walnuts

For dressing:

- ¼ cup fresh orange juice
- 1 tbsp minced red onion or shallot
- ½ tbsp agave nectar or maple syrup
- 2 tbsp olive oil
- 1 tbsp red wine vinegar
- Salt to taste

Directions:

1. Add black barley and water (if you are using any other grains, cook them according to the instructions given on the package) into a pot. Place the pot over high heat.
2. When it comes to a boil, lower the heat and cook covered until *al dente*. It can take about 45–60 minutes.
3. Meanwhile, add all the ingredients for the dressing into a bowl and whisk well.
4. Divide the barley equally into 2 bowls. Add similar quantities of the rest of the ingredients into the bowls, over the barley.
5. Pour dressing on top and serve.

Super Immune-Boosting Salad

Serves: 2–3

Ingredients:

- 4 medium beets, peeled, grated

- 2 in. fresh ginger, peeled, grated
- 8 large kale leaves, discard hard stem and ribs, chopped
- 2 tbsp hemp seed oil
- Sea salt to taste
- 2 large stalks celery, sliced
- 2 cloves garlic, minced, crushed
- 2 handfuls parsley, chopped
- 2 tbsp apple cider vinegar

Optional ingredients: Use any

- Nuts or seeds of your choice
- Hemp seeds
- Cooked or canned chickpeas
- Any other ingredients of your choice

Directions:

1. Add all the ingredients including optional ingredients into a large bowl. Toss well and serve.

Three Bean Salad

Serves: 3

Ingredients:

For salad:

- 1 celery stalk, chopped
- ½ cucumber, sliced
- ½ can (from a 15 oz can) chickpeas
- ½ can (from a 15 oz can) cannellini beans

- ½ can (from a 15 oz can) red kidney beans
- 1 small red onion, sliced
- ½ cup fresh parsley

For dressing:

- 2 tbsp red wine vinegar
- 1 tbsp water
- Salt to taste
- 1 tbsp maple syrup
- ½ tsp dried oregano
- Pepper to taste

Directions:

1. Add all the ingredients for salad into a bowl and toss well.
2. Add all the ingredients for dressing into a bowl and whisk well.
3. Pour the dressing over the salad. Toss well. Chill for a couple of hours and serve.

Coconut Ginger Carrot Soup

Serves: 2

Ingredients:

- 1 small white onion, diced
- 1 tbsp minced fresh ginger
- 2 ½ cup chopped carrot
- 2 cloves garlic, peeled, minced
- ½ tsp ground coriander
- ½ tsp ground cumin
- 1 ½ cup vegetable stock

- Salt to taste
- ½ cup full-fat coconut milk
- Pepper to taste
- 1 tsp olive oil

To serve:

- Lemon juice
- Chopped cilantro

Directions:

1. Place a soup pot over medium flame. Add oil. When the oil is heated, add onion and cook them until they're translucent.
2. Stir in carrot, ginger, garlic, cumin, and coriander and cook for a minute or so until fragrant.
3. Pour in broth and coconut milk and stir. Cook until carrots are soft. Blend with an immersion blender until smooth. Add salt and pepper to taste.
4. Ladle into soup bowls and drizzle with lemon juice. Garnish with cilantro and serve.

Immune-Boosting Soup

Serves: 3–4

Ingredients:

- ½ tbsp coconut oil
- 3 cloves garlic, minced
- ½ pound shiitake mushrooms, cut into large pieces
- Pepper to taste
- 6 cups water

- Salt to taste
- ½ tsp turmeric powder
- 2 heads baby Bok Choy, trim the bottoms
- ½ tbsp freshly grated ginger
- ½ large yellow onion, chopped
- 1 stalk celery, sliced
- 5–6 kale leaves, discard hard ribs and stems, chopped

Directions:

1. Place a soup pot over medium flame. Add oil. When the oil is heated, add onion and cook until pink.
2. Stir in the garlic and cook for a few seconds until fragrant.
3. Next add in the mushroom and celery and cook until the mushrooms are slightly cooked.
4. Add turmeric and ginger and stir for a few seconds. Add water and stir.
5. When it comes to a boil, lower the heat and cover with a lid. Cook for about 30 minutes.
6. Add Bok Choy and kale and cook until it wilts.
7. Ladle into soup bowls and serve hot.

Creamy Curried Cauliflower Lentil Soup

Serves: 2

Ingredients:

- 1 tsp avocado oil
- 1 medium carrot, diced
- ¾ tsp minced fresh ginger
- ½ head cauliflower, cut into bite size pieces

- Cayenne pepper to taste (optional)
- ¼ cup red lentils, rinsed
- 1 tbsp coconut cream
- ½ medium onion, chopped
- ½ stalk celery, diced
- 1 large clove garlic, minced
- 1–2 tsp curry powder
- 2 cup vegetable broth
- Salt to taste

Directions:

1. Place a soup pot over medium flame. Add oil. When the oil is heated, add onion, celery, and carrot and cook for a few minutes until the onion turns translucent.
2. Stir in the garlic and ginger and cook for about a minute.
3. Stir in cauliflower, lentils, salt, broth, and spices. When the soup comes to a boil, lower the heat and cook until the lentils are soft. Turn off the heat.
4. Add coconut cream and stir. Cool for a few minutes. Pour into a blender and blend until smooth. Heat if desired.
5. Ladle into soup bowls and enjoy!

Blueberry Quinoa Breakfast Bowl

Serves: 2

Ingredients:

For quinoa:

- ½ cup dry quinoa
- 1 ripe banana, sliced

- 1 cup water
- ½ cup frozen blueberries

For toppings: (optional)

- ½ tbsp maple syrup
- Almond milk, unsweetened, as required
- ½ tbsp chopped pecans or walnuts

Directions:

1. Add all the ingredients for quinoa into a saucepan. Place the saucepan over medium-low heat and cook covered, until dry.
2. Fluff with a fork.
3. Divide into 2 bowls. Add almond milk and stir. Drizzle maple syrup and sprinkle pecans on top before serving.

Sun-Dried Tomato and Kale Pasta

Serves: 3–4

Ingredients:

- 1 medium onion, chopped
- 1 tbsp tomato paste
- Pepper to taste
- 1 ¼ cup vegetable broth
- ½ pound whole grain penne pasta
- ¼ cup nutritional yeast
- 2 cloves garlic, minced
- Salt to taste
- 2 oz sun-dried tomatoes
- 1 ¼ cups unsweetened almond milk

- 2.5 oz kale, discard hard ribs and stems, chopped
- Crushed red pepper to garnish

Directions:

1. Place a nonstick pan over medium-high heat. Spray some cooking spray if desired or else add a tbsp of water. Add onion and cook until translucent.
2. Stir in the garlic and cook for a few seconds until fragrant.
3. Add tomato paste, salt and pepper, and mix well. Stir in the sun-dried tomatoes and cook for a couple of minutes.
4. Add milk and broth and stir. Cook on high. When it comes to a boil, stir in the pasta and lower the heat. Cook covered, until the pasta is nearly *al dente.*
5. Then, stir in the kale. Cook until the kale wilts. Stir in the nutritional yeast. Taste and adjust the seasoning if required and serve.

Mushroom Garlic Risotto

Serves: 2–3

Ingredients:

- ¾ cup short grain brown rice, rinsed, soaked in water for preferably 7–8 hours, drained
- 1 brown onion, chopped
- 3 cloves garlic, sliced
- 2 cups hot vegetable stock or 2 cup boiling water mixed with 2 vegetable stock cubes
- 2 ½ cup chopped spinach
- Pepper to taste

- ¼ cup kombucha
- 2 tbsp nutritional yeast
- Salt to taste
- 1 tbsp coconut oil
- 3 cup sliced mushrooms

To serve:

- Microgreens
- Olive oil

Directions:

1. Place a pot over medium flame. Add oil. When the oil is heated, add the onion and cook until they are pink.
2. Stir in the garlic and mushrooms and cook for a few minutes until the mushrooms are slightly brown.
3. Add rice and kombucha and cook until dry.
4. Pour ½ cup broth and cook until dry, on low heat.
5. Repeat the previous step until all the broth is added. Once all the broth is added the rice should be cooked.
6. Stir in nutritional yeast, salt, spinach, and pepper and cook until the spinach wilts.
7. Serve risotto topped with micro greens and olive oil.

Stuffed Bell Peppers

Serves: 2–3

Ingredients:

- 2–3 large bell peppers, use any color of your choice, cut off a slice from the tops, and deseed

- 2 cloves garlic, minced
- ½ cup frozen corn
- ½ cup cooked brown rice
- ½ bunch cilantro, chopped
- ½ yellow onion, finely chopped
- 1 chipotle pepper in adobo sauce, minced
- ½ can (from a 15 oz can) black beans, drained, rinsed
- ½ can (from a 14 oz can) diced tomatoes, drained
- Salt to taste
- Pepper to taste

For toppings: (optional)

- Cashew sour cream
- Crushed tortilla chips
- Green onion, sliced

Directions:

1. Place a pot filled with water over high heat and bring to a boil.
2. Drop the bell peppers in the boiling water and cook for about 3 minutes or until slightly soft. Drain the water and remove any moisture that is in the peppers. Place them in a baking dish.
3. Place a nonstick pan over medium heat. Add onion and about a tbsp of water and cook until soft.
4. Stir in garlic, corn, chipotle pepper and black beans. Heat thoroughly. Transfer into a bowl.
5. Add cilantro, brown rice, and tomatoes and mix well. Fill this mixture into the bell peppers.
6. Bake in a preheated oven at 350 °F for about 30–40 minutes. Top with tortilla chips, cashew sour cream, and green onions and serve.

PB & Beets Sandwich

Serves: 4

Ingredients:

- 4 slices whole wheat bread, toasted
- ½ cup MamaSezz Strong Heart Beats
- ½ cup natural peanut butter

Directions:

1. Apply peanut butter on the bread slices.
2. Spread Strong Heart Beats over the slices and serve.

Garlic Ginger Broccoli

Serves: 4–6

Ingredients:

- 2 heads broccoli, cut into bite size florets
- 2 tbsp minced ginger
- 4 tbsp agave nectar
- 2 tbsp sesame seeds
- 4 cloves garlic, peeled, minced
- 4 tbsp tamari
- 2 tbsp chili paste or more to taste

Directions:

1. Place a skillet over medium heat. Add 2–3 tbsp of water and add broccoli. Stir often and cook until broccoli is bright green in color. Sprinkle more water if required while cooking.
2. Move the broccoli to the edges of the pan and add ginger and garlic in the center. Cook for a couple of minutes until aromatic.
3. Move the broccoli back to the center and mix well. Add remaining ingredients and continue combining. Heat thoroughly and serve.

Chocolate Covered Strawberries

Serves: 6

Ingredients:

- 6 fresh strawberries
- 3 dates, pitted, soaked in water for about an hour, drained
- A pinch salt
- ⅛ cup cashews, soaked in water for 4–5 hours, drained
- ½ tbsp cacao powder
- Water, as required

Directions:

1. Place strawberries in a bowl.
2. Add dates, salt, cashews, cacao powder and water into a blender and blend until smooth.
3. Pour over the strawberries.
4. Take 6 bowls. Place a strawberry in each. Drizzle sauce over it and serve.

Conclusion

Now you can see that a plant-based diet is extremely simple to follow and offers a variety of benefits. These benefits are not just restricted to improving your health, but you can help the environment, too. This simple diet is an all-around winning choice. The plant-based diet is certainly superior to eating meat. The meat industry not only indulges in unethical practices, but it is downright inhumane to the animals involved. Instead of treating them as sentient beings, they are used as a living food source. Humans have farmed animals for thousands of years, but this became a rampant problem in the last couple of decades—your decision to go forward with plant-based alternatives will help put an end to it.

To keep up with the ever-increasing demand for meat, the meat industry started pumping the animals with antibiotics, growth hormones and cramping them into tightly-packed areas to save space and increase production. The various statistics mentioned in this book are chilling and unsettling. However, they introduce us to the reality of the meat industry and motivate us all to make changes.

By following a plant-based diet, you get all the nutrients your body needs, and you get them ethically. Instead of sending innocent animals to the slaughter, your nourishment comes from healthy plants. If you are ever worried about needing any additional supplements, go through the list of supplements given in this book, and try adding as many of those nutritious ingredients as you possibly can. A plant-based diet can help you lose and maintain weight, improve your heart's health, reduce the risk of diabetes, certain types of cancers, while aiding the environment's recovery.

A plant-based diet is ethical, unlike the unethical reality of the cruel treatment that animal agriculture requires. Not only does it spread diseases, but the commercial production of cheap meat and various animal products is unethical, inhumane, and cruel. Several environmental issues stem from animal farming. From pollution of precious natural resources to greenhouse gas emissions, deforestation, and soil disruption, the negative effects of cheap animal farming cannot be overlooked anymore. The need of the hour is to explore sustainable alternatives to animal farming. All the resources used by animal farming can be used to produce plant-based foods. This simple solution has the potential to end world hunger and prevent subjecting innocent animals to a miserable existence.

There is an undeniable link between meat and animal products' consumption and several pandemics. From the first mad cow outbreak in 1986 to the latest coronavirus outbreak in 2020, these pandemics are caused by using animal products. Of course wearing a mask, using a sanitizer, and practicing social distancing has become the norm, but it doesn't have to be this way. Imagine the kind of world we are leaving behind for our children and future generations. The simplest way to protect yourself from any such trouble in the future is to eliminate meat. It is a simple change that results in priceless benefits for everyone.

In the course of this book, you got a detailed plant-based food list for following a plant-based diet. By adding wholesome and healthy plant-based foods and eliminating all sorts of animal products from your daily diet, you can improve your overall health. Following this diet is not only simple, but it is sustainable in the long run too. It is not a fad diet and is instead a holistic lifestyle change. Follow the simple and practical tips given in this book to transition to a new plant-based lifestyle smoothly.

You've also learned a wide array of easy plant-based recipes. These recipes are not only simple to follow but also extremely nutritious and delicious. The ingredients used in these recipes are all simple plant-based ingredients, which are easily available in your local farmers market. For better results, use as much organic produce as possible, it will not just be good for your health, but will also elevate the taste of your dishes. Cooking tasty and healthy food has never been this simple.

Once you start following the plant-based diet, you are essentially eating your way to a healthier and more sustainable lifestyle. To get used to this new diet, review and follow the expertly crafted tips and techniques given in this book. Remember, it will take your body some time to get used to the new diet. In the meanwhile, believe in the process and the diet, and be patient with yourself. Once you start following this diet, you will notice a favorable change in your overall fitness and health. Whenever you feel a little low on motivation, remind yourself of all the good you are doing. This simple change on a personal level has global implications. Never give up on this diet, and always keep going. Now, all that's left for you to do is start following the advice in this book, and get accustomed to this new way of life.

Now that you've reached the end of the book, I hope you enjoyed reading it as much as I did while writing. If you liked this book, please leave a review!

Thank you!

References

Alena, & Lars. (2015, October 8). Nutriciously - Healthy Plant-Based Eating. Retrieved from nutritiously website: https://nutriciously.com/

Alena. (2016, September 25). The 22 Best Vegan Documentaries to Inspire You. Retrieved from nutritiously website: https://nutriciously.com/best-vegan-documentaries/

Alena. (2019, September 10). 12 Tips on How to Start a Plant-Based Diet. Retrieved from nutritiously website: https://nutriciously.com/start-a-plant-based-diet/

Altekruse, S. F., Timbo, B. B., Mowbray, J. C., Bean, N. H., & Potter, M. E. (1998). Cheese-associated outbreaks of human illness in the United States, 1973 to 1992: sanitary manufacturing practices protect consumers. *Journal of Food Protection, 61*(10), 1405–1407. https://doi.org/10.4315/0362-028x-61.10.1405

Anthis, J. R. (2017). Survey of US Attitudes Towards Animal Farming and Animal-Free Food. *Www.Sentience Institute.Org.* Retrieved from https://www.sentienceinstitute.org/animal-farming-attitudes-survey-2017

Bar-On, Y. M., Phillips, R., & Milo, R. (2018). The biomass distribution on Earth. *Proceedings of the National Academy of Sciences, 115*(25), 6506–6511. https://doi.org/10.1073/pnas.1711842115

Barr, S., & Wright, J. (2010). Postprandial energy expenditure in whole-food and processed-food meals: implications for daily energy expenditure. *Food & Nutrition Research, 54*(1), 5144. https://doi.org/10.3402/fnr.v54i0.5144

Blom, W. A., Lluch, A., Stafleu, A., Vinoy, S., Holst, J. J., Schaafsma, G., & Hendriks, H. F. (2006). Effect of a high-protein breakfast on the postprandial ghrelin response. *The American Journal of Clinical Nutrition*, *83*(2), 211–220. https://doi.org/10.1093/ajcn/83.2.211

Brown, S. (2019, April 29). How livestock farming affects the environment. Retrieved from www.downtoearth.org.in website: https://www.downtoearth.org.in/factsheet/how-livestock-farming-affects-the-environment-64218#:~:text=Raising%20livestock%20generates%2014.5%20per

Burdge, G. C., Tan, S. Y., & Henry, C. J. (2017). Long-chain *n*-3 PUFA in vegetarian women: a metabolic perspective. *Journal of nutritional science*, *6*, e58. https://doi.org/10.1017/jns.2017.62

Cameron, J., & Suzy Amis Cameron. (2018, August 9). Animal agriculture is choking the Earth and making us sick. We must act now | James Cameron and Suzy Amis Cameron. Retrieved from the Guardian website: https://www.theguardian.com/commentisfree/2017/dec/04/animal-agriculture-choking-earth-making-sick-climate-food-environmental-impact-james-cameron-suzy-amis-cameron

Cassidy, E. S., West, P. C., Gerber, J. S., & Foley, J. A. (2013). Redefining agricultural yields: from tonnes to people nourished per hectare. *Environmental Research Letters*, *8*(3), 034015. https://doi.org/10.1088/1748-9326/8/3/034015

Chan, J. M., & Giovannucci, E. L. (2001). Dairy products, calcium, and vitamin D and risk of prostate cancer. *Epidemiologic reviews*, *23*(1), 87–92. https://doi.org/10.1093/oxfordjournals.epirev.a000800

Chuang, S.-Y., Chiu, T. H. T., Lee, C.-Y., Liu, T.-T., Tsao, C. K., Hsiung, C. A., & Chiu, Y.-F. (2016). Vegetarian diet reduces the risk of hypertension independent of abdominal obesity and inflammation: a prospective study. *Journal of Hypertension*, *34*(11), 2164–2171. https://doi.org/10.1097/HJH.0000000000001068

Clarys, P., Deliens, T., Huybrechts, I., Deriemaeker, P., Vanaelst, B., De Keyzer, W., … Mullie, P. (2014). Comparison of Nutritional Quality of the Vegan, Vegetarian, Semi-Vegetarian, Pesco-Vegetarian and Omnivorous Diet. *Nutrients*, *6*(3), 1318–1332. https://doi.org/10.3390/nu6031318

Climate Change and Animal Agriculture, Explained | PETA. (2015, April 29). Retrieved from PETA website: https://www.peta.org/features/climate-change-animal-agriculture-explained/

Dahl-Jørgensen, K., Joner, G., & Hanssen, K. F. (1991). Relationship between cows' milk consumption and incidence of IDDM in childhood. *Diabetes Care*, *14*(11), 1081–1083. https://doi.org/10.2337/diacare.14.11.1081

Dunphy, S. (2019, October 29). Eating a healthy diet could reduce environmental impacts. Retrieved from European Scientist website: https://www.europeanscientist.com/en/public-health/eating-a-healthy-diet-could-reduce-environmental-impacts/

Foster, M., Chu, A., Petocz, P., & Samman, S. (2013). Effect of vegetarian diets on zinc status: a systematic review and meta-analysis of studies in humans. *Journal of the Science of Food and Agriculture*, *93*(10), 2362–2371. https://doi.org/10.1002/jsfa.6179

Gerstein, H. C. (1994). Cow's Milk Exposure and Type I Diabetes Mellitus: A critical overview of the clinical literature. *Diabetes Care*, *17*(1), 13–19. https://doi.org/10.2337/diacare.17.1.13

Hever, J. (2016). Plant-Based Diets: A Physician's Guide. *The Permanente Journal*. https://doi.org/10.7812/tpp/15-082

Hill, A., RDN, & LD. (2020, February 21). The 4 Main Types of Plant-Based Diets. Retrieved from Clean Green Simple website: https://cleangreensimple.com/article/types-of-plant-based-diets/

Horrigan, L., Lawrence, R. S., & Walker, P. (2002). How sustainable agriculture can address the environmental and human health harms of industrial agriculture. *Environmental Health Perspectives*, *110*(5), 445–456. Retrieved from http://www.ncbi.nlm.nih.gov/pmc/articles/PMC1240832/

How much does animal agriculture and eating meat contribute to global warming? (2019). Retrieved from Skeptical Science website: https://skepticalscience.com/animal-agriculture-meat-global-warming.htm

Kim, H., Caulfield, L. E., & Rebholz, C. M. (2018). Healthy Plant-Based Diets Are Associated with Lower Risk of All-Cause Mortality in US Adults. *The Journal of Nutrition*, *148*(4), 624–631. https://doi.org/10.1093/jn/nxy019

Kim, H., Caulfield, L. E., Garcia-Larsen, V., Steffen, L. M., Coresh, J., & Rebholz, C. M. (2019). Plant-Based Diets Are Associated With a Lower Risk of Incident Cardiovascular Disease, Cardiovascular Disease Mortality, and All-Cause Mortality in a General Population of Middle-Aged Adults. *Journal of the American Heart Association*, *8*(16). https://doi.org/10.1161/jaha.119.012865

Link, R. (2017, July 28). 12 Mistakes to Avoid on a Vegetarian or Vegan Diet. Retrieved from Healthline website: https://www.healthline.com/nutrition/vegetarian-and-vegan-mistakes#section13

Marino, L., & Allen, K. (2017). The Psychology of Cows. *Animal Behavior and Cognition*, *4*(4), 474–498. https://doi.org/10.26451/abc.04.04.06.2017

Maruyama, K., Oshima, T., & Ohyama, K. (2010). Exposure to exogenous estrogen through intake of commercial milk produced from pregnant cows. *Pediatrics International: Official Journal of the Japan Pediatric Society*, *52*(1), 33–38. https://doi.org/10.1111/j.1442-200X.2009.02890.x

Matteo, A. (2015, January 6). Western Diet Bad for Human Health, Environment. Retrieved from VOA website: https://learningenglish.voanews.com/a/western-diet-bad-for-human-health-environment/2579378.html

McMahon, J. (2019, April 4). Meat And Agriculture Are Worse For The Climate Than Power Generation, Steven Chu Says. Retrieved from Forbes website: https://www.forbes.com/sites/jeffmcmahon/2019/04/04/meat-and-agriculture-are-worse-for-the-climate-than-dirty-energy-steven-chu-says/#21e8ed1311f9

More Reasons to Go Vegan | PETA. (2010, July 16). Retrieved from PETA website: https://www.peta.org/issues/animals-used-for-food/reasons-go-vegan/

Multistate Outbreak of Listeriosis Linked to Blue Bell Creameries Products| Listeria | CDC. (2018, December 3). Retrieved from www.cdc.gov website: http://www.cdc.gov/listeria/outbreaks/ice-cream-03-15

Nicole, W. (2013). CAFOs and Environmental Justice: The Case of North Carolina. *Environmental Health Perspectives*, *121*(6). https://doi.org/10.1289/ehp.121-a182

PETA Prime: New Study: Go Vegan and Help End World Hunger. (2013, August 20). Retrieved from PETA Prime website: https://prime.peta.org/2013/08/hunger/

Plourde, M., & Cunnane, S. C. (2007). Extremely limited synthesis of long chain polyunsaturates in adults: implications for their dietary essentiality and use as supplements. *Applied Physiology,*

Nutrition, and Metabolism = Physiologie Appliquee, Nutrition Et Metabolisme, *32*(4), 619–634. https://doi.org/10.1139/H07-034

Rose, C. (2012, April 10). The Greenest Act: A Plant-based Diet. Retrieved from Down to Earth Organic and Natural website: https://www.downtoearth.org/articles/2012-04/2793/greenest-act-plant-based-diet#:~:text=Switching%20from%20a%20meat%2Dbased

Satija, A., Bhupathiraju, S. N., Rimm, E. B., Spiegelman, D., Chiuve, S. E., Borgi, L., … Hu, F. B. (2016). Plant-Based Dietary Patterns and Incidence of Type 2 Diabetes in US Men and Women: Results from Three Prospective Cohort Studies. *PLOS Medicine*, *13*(6), e1002039. https://doi.org/10.1371/journal.pmed.1002039

Saunders, A. V., Craig, W. J., Baines, S. K., & Posen, J. S. (2013). Iron and vegetarian diets. *The Medical Journal of Australia*, *199*(S4), S11–16. Retrieved from https://pubmed.ncbi.nlm.nih.gov/25369923/

Tilman, D., & Clark, M. (2014). Global diets link environmental sustainability and human health. *Nature*, *515*(7528), 518–522. https://doi.org/10.1038/nature13959

Tonstad, S., Butler, T., Yan, R., & Fraser, G. E. (2009). Type of Vegetarian Diet, Body Weight, and Prevalence of Type 2 Diabetes. *Diabetes Care*, *32*(5), 791–796. https://doi.org/10.2337/dc08-1886

Ventrice, M. (2020, January 2). 5 Ways Eating More Plant-Based Foods Benefits the Environment. Retrieved from One Green Planet website: https://www.onegreenplanet.org/environment/how-eating-more-plant-based-foods-benefits-the-environment/

Watanabe, F., Yabuta, Y., Bito, T., & Teng, F. (2014). Vitamin B12-Containing Plant Food Sources for Vegetarians. *Nutrients*, *6*(5), 1861–1873. https://doi.org/10.3390/nu6051861

Weinsier, R. L., & Krumdieck, C. L. (2000). Dairy foods and bone health: examination of the evidence. *The American Journal of Clinical Nutrition*, *72*(3), 681–689. https://doi.org/10.1093/ajcn/72.3.681

Wright, N., Wilson, L., Smith, M., Duncan, B., & McHugh, P. (2017). The BROAD study: A randomised controlled trial using a whole food plant-based diet in the community for obesity, ischaemic heart disease or diabetes. *Nutrition & Diabetes*, *7*(3), e256. https://doi.org/10.1038/nutd.2017.3

Yokoyama, Y., Nishimura, K., Barnard, N. D., Takegami, M., Watanabe, M., Sekikawa, A., … Miyamoto, Y. (2014). Vegetarian Diets and Blood Pressure. *JAMA Internal Medicine*, *174*(4), 577. https://doi.org/10.1001/jamainternmed.2013.14547

Zuñiga, Y. L. M., Rebello, S. A., Oi, P. L., Zheng, H., Lee, J., Tai, E. S., & Van Dam, R. M. (2014). Rice and noodle consumption is associated with insulin resistance and hyperglycemia in an Asian population. *The British Journal of Nutrition*, *111*(6), 1118–1128. https://doi.org/10.1017/S0007114513003486

www.ingramcontent.com/pod-product-compliance
Lightning Source LLC
LaVergne TN
LVHW020628100826
845148LV00012B/2097

* 9 7 8 1 7 3 6 8 2 0 5 1 3 *